Stroke affects the personal, social, professional ar[...]
their carers. This book is based on a study in which 173 stroke patients and their
family carers were followed from the time of the stroke for a period of eighteen
months. It tells of their experience of the illness and examines their patterns of
coping, including physical, social, economic and emotional aspects.

The words of the patients and their carers illuminate these histories of life after
stroke, vividly expressing the difficulties encountered with the services designed to
help them. At a time when the health and welfare services in many countries are
rethinking their strategies for community care, this study underlines the importance of social factors in recovery after stroke.

Written for all health care professionals involved with stroke patients, this
careful and comprehensive account will direct attention to practices which
can improve the quality of life for people with chronic illness, and their carers.

The Aftermath of *Stroke*

The Aftermath of *Stroke*

The experience of patients and their families

ROBERT ANDERSON

Formerly Senior Research Officer
Institute for Social Studies in Medical Care, London

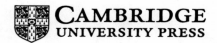

CAMBRIDGE
UNIVERSITY PRESS

CAMBRIDGE UNIVERSITY PRESS
Cambridge, New York, Melbourne, Madrid, Cape Town, Singapore, São Paulo

Cambridge University Press
The Edinburgh Building, Cambridge CB2 2RU, UK

Published in the United States of America by Cambridge University Press, New York

www.cambridge.org
Information on this title: www.cambridge.org/9780521401968

First published 1992
This digitally printed first paperback version 2006

A catalogue record for this publication is available from the British Library

Library of Congress Cataloguing in Publication data
Anderson, Robert, 1944–
The aftermath of stroke: the experience of patients and
their families/Robert Anderson.
p.   cm.
Includes bibliographical references and index.
ISBN 0 521 40196 8 (hardback)
1. Cerebrovascular disease – Patients – Rehabilitation.
2. Cerebrovascular disease – Patients – Family relationships.
3. Cerebrovascular disease – Psychological aspects.   I. Title.
[DNLM: 1. Cerebrovascular Disorders – psychology.
2. Cerebrovascular Disorders – rehabilitation.
3. Family – psychology.   4. Social Support. WL 355 A549a]
RC388.5.A535   1992
362.1'9681–dc20   91-29397   CIP

ISBN-13 978-0-521-40196-8 hardback
ISBN-10 0-521-40196-8 hardback   NOV   2007

ISBN-13 978-0-521-02982-7 paperback
ISBN-10 0-521-02982-1 paperback

Contents

Acknowledgements

Many people have helped and contributed to the study reported here, but foremost are the stroke patients and their supporters, who gave so much time to me and to Sue Tester, who interviewed all the main supporters over a period of two and a half years. I am greatly indebted to the skill and sensitivity with which Sue Tester interviewed supporters, and to the same qualities that Ann Buxton showed in her interviews with general practitioners. As a social scientist I have been in particular need of help from people whose work involves them in the rehabilitation, care and support of stroke patients and their families: the advisory group of Rachel David, Anne Dummett, Meg Holbrook, David Mulhall, Annemarie Tupper and Jean Weddell; people in Greenwich health district who supported and helped to develop the study: Mohammed Ali, Yvonne Bacchus, Peter Blower, Carole Brooker, May Clarke, Stephen Fash, Philip Marsden, Ged Moran, Jackie Mugford, William Nicholson, D. O'Connor, Helen Ransome, Rosalinde Recardo, Tony Ruffell and Lorna Stewart; and staff in rehabilitation and other services who provided advice and support: Rosemary Barnitt, Jayne Comins, Christine Diebel, Pat Farnham, Jean Tarling, Sue Toller, Derick Wade and Jo Willinson.

The detailed checking of the analyses and their interpretation was done with skill and patience by Joy Windsor. Joe Bolton provided extensive support in preparing the data and computing, with help from Danny Kushlick and Polly Wilson. I am grateful, too, for coding by Dorothy Goodwin and Margaret Hall; for help with preparation of the manuscript by Charlotte Harrison, Nichola Schild and Heather Taylor; and for photocopying by Emma and Lucy Jefferys. For advice and support I am particularly grateful to Ann Cartwright, to other former colleagues at the Institute for Social Studies in Medical Care, London: Ann Jacoby, Madeleine Simms and Chris Smith; and to members of the Institute's Advisory Committee: Abe Adelstein, Tony Alment, Val Beral, Vera

Carstairs, Karen Dunnell, Austin Heady, Margot Jefferys, Joyce Leeson, John McEwan, Martin Richards, Alwyn Smith and Mike Wadsworth.

The study was funded by the Department of Health and Social Security, and benefited from the help and support of Doreen Rothman and Marguerite Smith. Finally, I am grateful to all the general practitioners, consultants, practice managers and receptionists, and hospital nurses, who helped to establish the community register on which the study was based.

Most of these people have influenced the development and outcome of this study, but of course only I am responsible for the views expressed here.

Monkstown   Robert Anderson

CHAPTER ONE

Stroke: An introduction to the problem

Every year, in a typical Western population of 100 000 people, about 200 suffer a stroke and come into medical care. Most of these people are admitted to hospital but the proportion varies, depending, in part, upon whether the patient lives in town or country. Stroke is the most important single cause of hospital use after mental disorders; altogether, care of stroke patients may absorb about 6% of hospital running costs and nearly 5% of all National Health Service costs (Carstairs, 1976). As a report from the Royal College of Physicians (1990) underlines, stroke is a major cause of chronic disability and the source of a heavy burden on patients' relatives and friends, as well as consuming a great deal of the resources of the health and welfare services.

About a quarter of the people who suffer a stroke die in the first month, but more than half survive for a year or more (Aho et al., 1980; Warlow et al., 1987). Most stroke survivors, probably about two-thirds, are rated as independent in daily activities by 1 year after the stroke (Weddell and Beresford, 1979; Wade et al., 1985b; Warlow et al., 1987), although this does not mean that they have returned to levels of activity or performance that they had before the stroke. Altogether, in a population of 100 000 people there are roughly 750 survivors of stroke, most of them living in the community with, or near to, family, and with varying levels of disability (Warlow et al., 1987).

On the basis of existing research it is possible to describe quite well the characteristics of the people who suffer a stroke; which of them survive, and for how long; the ways in which they are dependent on others; which patients make improvements in physical functioning; and which of them return home. These themes – the factors that influence medical management and rehabilitation – reflect the principal concerns of most investigators. A broader perspective, including social aspects of stroke and follow-up over time in the community, is given in some recent studies (esp. Wade, 1984). However, the effects of stroke on family relationships, housing, money, social life and general attitudes to life has been relatively neglected. Even less so, has research considered the perspectives – the views, attitudes and preferences – of patients and their family supporters, either alone or in relation to each other. Little is known about how patients and supporters feel about the care and support they receive; about how they want to be helped and what information they require; about which problems distress them most; or about how they view the main effects of stroke on their lives.

The experience of a chronic illness such as stroke, and its implications for practice, cannot be reduced to the rise and fall of performance in activities of daily living. There is a need to make policies and services relevant to the everyday lives of people living in the community. The effects of stroke on everyday life can be considered within the framework developed by Wood (1980) and discussed as handicaps (see Bury, 1987); while disability refers to loss of the ability to perform an activity, handicap refers to the disadvantage that accrues from being unable to fulfil a role that is normal for that individual. Thus the nature of disadvantage will depend upon social values and culture, but people will generally be disadvantaged if they are unable to orient themselves, move around, manage their body's physical needs, occupy time with work or recreation, maintain social relationships and be economically self-sufficient. These accomplishments constitute the core dimensions of handicap (Wood, 1980) and provide the framework for the discussion of the experience of stroke presented here.

The dimensions of handicap can be considered just as readily for family carers as for patients, and that is also done here. When stroke is dealt with as a 'family illness' the permutations of 'successful' recovery increase in number; there has been almost no research into the influence of the perspectives and perceptions of patients and their carers on the process of recovery from the stroke. Assessments of outcome have typically been made in terms relevant to the goals of the many professions involved; apart from the biographies of strong-willed and resourceful individuals there is no systematic information on the meaning of the stroke for patients and their carers. Yet if services are to support patients and their carers there is a need for greater awareness of the experiences and views of the main parties involved.

This book reports a study of the experience of a stroke as seen from the perspectives of patients and their main supporters. It looks at who provided what help, and what happened to whom, but it is mainly concerned with changes in the daily lives and attitudes of patients and supporters over the first 18 months after a stroke. When patients survive the first weeks after a stroke they and their families embark upon a complex process of change and accommodation. This may lead to major changes in lifestyle, not only in patterns of social activities, housing, family relationships and financial circumstances but also in values, expectations and priorities. The perception and meaning of life may be altered. The chapters that follow aim to increase awareness and understanding of this process of change following stroke.

The meaning of stroke and the response to disability depend upon access to different elements in the 'armoury of resources' (Croog and Levine, 1977) – systems of personal, informal, community and institutional support. Evidently these resources are not distributed equally among people (with or without chronic illness) but may vary with sex, social class and age (Locker, 1983). These three characteristics will be investigated throughout the report as core variables influencing response to stroke and disability. Among the social resources for patients and their families, the health and social services are major supports upon which people may draw. Their contribution is considered in terms of their availability, the attitudes of patients and their supporters, and the effects of services on changes in the lives of patients and their supporters. In the context of viewing the stroke as a family illness with diverse and long-term consequences for the lives of patients and their supporters, it is important to identify gaps in service provision. There is currently widespread discussion of services which are relevant to the whole person, which improve quality of life, and which support the supporters. What is offered here is an opportunity to locate the rhetoric in the reality of life after a stroke.

Any attempt to review and assimilate the existing research literature is fraught with difficulties, the principal one being that much of the research with stroke patients is neither comparable nor cumulative. Studies of stroke patients are often conducted with small, convenient groups, and the sample populations vary in characteristics such as the definition of stroke used, age, degree of initial disability, management in home, hospital or rehabilitation centre, time since onset of the stroke, and measures of outcome or recovery. Major studies with which authors often compare their own results have included men only (Baker *et al.*, 1968), hospital patients only (Marquardsen, 1969), hemiplegic patients only (Adams and Merrett, 1961) or those with hemiparesis (Brocklehurst *et al.*, 1978a), and those suffering transient ischaemic attacks (Wolf *et al.*, 1977). These constraints on comparisons are often not acknowledged, to say nothing of differences between studies in their methods (for example, the definition and validation of the diagnosis of stroke).

In part, the problem with definitions of stroke is that the term 'stroke' refers to a description of symptoms and signs rather than to a single underlying pathology. However, most of the more recent epidemiological studies in England and Wales (Chin *et al.*, 1980; Stevens and Ambler, 1982; Oxfordshire Community Stroke Project (OCSP), 1983; Wade and Langton-Hewer, 1985) have used the definition of stroke recommended by the World Health Organization (WHO); this was also used in the study reported here.

Incidence of stroke

European studies using prospective stroke registers have produced incidence rates of about 200 new cases of stroke every year in a population of 100 000 (Radic *et al.*, 1977; Herman *et al.*, 1980; OCSP, 1983). All studies show that stroke happens overwhelmingly to older people: in the studies from areas in England (OCSP, 1983; Wade *et al.*, 1985a; Stevens and Ambler, 1982) between 75% and 86% of stroke patients were aged 65 and over. In these prospective studies, between 55% and 60% of the initial sample of stroke patients have been women. This is not surprising given the relationship between age and incidence. However, there is some indication that, at least in certain age groups, men are more likely to have a stroke: in the studies from Carlisle (Chin *et al.*, 1980), Dover (Stevens and Ambler, 1982) and Farnham (Weddell and Beresford, 1979) there is a higher incidence among men aged 55 to 75; in Oxfordshire the greatest excess was among men aged 45 to 65, and the overall excess of risk of stroke among men was 30% (Warlow *et al.*, 1987) – a figure also estimated by Haberman and colleagues (1981) from a worldwide review of community and hospital-based studies.

There appears to be no published information on the relationship between social class or socio-economic status and the incidence of stroke; in the Farnham district study no link was found (J. Weddell, personal communication). The analysis of 'standard consulting ratios' in general practice reveals no social class trends – for men at least; the data are not presented for all women (Royal College of General Practitioners, 1982). Lack of a relationship between stroke incidence and social class would be surprising, given that in England and Wales there is a clear pattern of increasing mortality due to stroke with increasing social class (Evans, 1979). However, the nature of the relationship between stroke incidence and social or economic conditions has attracted little specific research.

Survival after stroke

The natural history of stroke involves a fairly high level of deaths soon after the stroke, followed by a lower but relatively continuous fatality over succeeding years. The aggregated data from the WHO study (Aho *et al.*, 1980), in which there were no significant differences in survival rates between centres, showed 23% dying within 7 days, 31% within 3 weeks and 48% before the end of the first year after a stroke. The figures are similar in reports of other studies, suggesting that, on average, half or more of all stroke patients survive beyond 1 year. Survival in two English studies, which were also organised along the lines of the WHO study, appear rather worse than average: preliminary results from Carlisle (Chin *et al.*, 1980) show 54% of patients died in the first month, while in Farnham (Weddell and Beresford, 1979) 54% of patients died in the first 3 months. However, results from the Oxfordshire study, which appears to have good coverage of milder cases of stroke, indicate that the overall 1-year case fatality rate is between 30% and 40% (Warlow *et al.*, 1987).

Most studies report that survival is more likely among younger patients (Ford and Katz, 1966; Aho *et al.*, 1980; Warlow *et al.*, 1987). However, a conspicuous feature of many different studies is the lack of any consistent relationship between sex and survival. There are few reports which consider other social characteristics of patients in relation to survival. In their study Abu-Zeid and colleagues (1978) found that, after adjusting for age, married patients were more likely to survive the stroke than single people. The same authors reported no association between stroke survival and socio-economic group, but Sussman (1965) refers to work, now more than 25 years old, showing that stroke patients with higher levels of economic dependence deteriorated more rapidly in their functioning and died sooner than less economically dependent patients.

In general, it appears that 'Irrespective of treatment, about a third of all stroke patients die of the condition, and the majority of these deaths occur very early' (Wright and Robson, 1980, p. 250). Among those who survive the acute stroke, subsequent mortality is almost certainly higher than in the general population of the same age and sex (Abu-Zeid *et al.*, 1978; Sacco *et al.*, 1982). About a quarter of survivors at 3 weeks may die before the end of the first year; thereafter deaths appear to progress at a rate of about 15% of the at-risk population every year. This is broadly compatible with the results from Farnham, where about 40% survived for between 3 weeks to 4 years after the stroke (Weddell and Beresford, 1979). There is a lack of detailed data on the longer-term survival of stroke patients, and the factors influencing this survival.

Consequences of stroke

In a limited sense, and subject to caveats about whether it is possible to generalise the results of different studies, there is a good deal of information about some consequences of the illness for both patients and their supporters.

Neurological impairment

The main symptoms of stroke vary, but frequently involve some period of unconsciousness, which may last for moments, hours or days. On recovering consciousness the patient commonly has one or more of the following difficulties: paralysis of one side of the body (hemiplegia); slighter loss of strength in one arm and one leg (hemiparesis); loss of feeling in, or loss of awareness of, the affected side of the body; weakness on one side of the face; difficulty in seeing out of one side of each eye; difficulty in understanding what is said and in speaking to others; difficulty in coughing or swallowing; and incontinence of bowel or bladder. Some of these deficits are associated with each other, due to the site or nature of the neurological lesion. Thus patients with weakness or paralysis on the left side of their body (left hemiplegia) more often have visuo-spatial and perceptual difficulties; patients with right hemiplegia are more likely to suffer from impairments in communication, particularly speech (dysphasia) (Adams, 1974; Brocklehurst *et al.*, 1978a).

Some evidence of weakness or paralysis has been found in between two-thirds (Stevens and Ambler, 1982) and five-sixths (Weddell and Beresford, 1979) of patients soon after the stroke. However, the proportion of survivors with limb weakness or paralysis declines through death and recovery, so that, for example, more than half of the survivors in the WHO multicentre study (Aho *et al.*, 1980) were free of hemiplegia or hemiparesis at 1 year after the stroke. It is against this general background that the consequent 'disability' or 'handicap' (Wood, 1980; Bury, 1987) can be described.

Disability and handicap

The patient's physical disability and dependence have been investigated more extensively than other consequences of stroke, although the meaning of disability in terms of disadvantage is seldom explicit. The ability to perform activities of daily living, often described as 'independence', does not necessarily mean 'back to normal'; patients may be able to walk 50 metres outdoors but be unable to reach the shops, to carry the shopping or work out how much the shopping cost.

Progress in performing activities of daily living slows after the first month, and appears to be virtually complete by about 6 months after the stroke (Brocklehurst *et al.*, 1978a). After 3 months nearly three-quarters of the survivors in Farnham were classified as independent in ability to get in or out of a chair; 1 in 30 was totally dependent. The ability of survivors 4 years after the stroke was similar (Weddell and Beresford, 1979). However, another survey, of the spouses of young (under age 65) survivors at least 3 years after the stroke, found that two-thirds of the patients were described by their family as having problems with self-care (Coughlan and Humphrey, 1982). This points to the difference between measurement of dependency and the experience or perception of difficulties by patients and their families.

The problem of communication between the patient and others may also be underestimated if conclusions are based solely on tests for dysphasia (i.e. capacity for interpretation and formulation of the symbols of communication). There is little doubt that impairment of the abilities to read, write, speak and understand are often found after a stroke; the frequency with which these disorders are reported depends upon the methods of assessment, the characteristics of the patients and the time since onset of the stroke at which assessments are made (Wade *et al.*, 1986b).

The spouses and chief carers of the stroke patients may identify problems in communication even though the patient has not been assessed as dysphasic (Artes and Hoops, 1976). At 1 month after the stroke, 39% of chief carers reported difficulties understanding the patient's speech in one study (Brocklehurst *et al.*, 1978a) while, in the longer-term, 1 in 4 spouses continued to report communication difficulties (Coughlan and Humphrey, 1982). Clearly, the experience of difficulties in communication is made up from more elements than ratings of clarity of expression or comprehension.

For patients, the experience of loss of the ability to communicate effectively means more than an inability to read or make clear requests: it is a cause of significant distress. Hurwitz and Adams (1972) note how frustrating dysphasia can be: 'being regarded as brainless, being subjected to the indignity of having things done for them which they could well do for themselves, and ... not doing for them those things they cannot possibly be expected to do' (p. 94). Anxiety and depression, even a sense of hopelessness, are found among a large number of all stroke victims, but 'The failure to be able to remember, to use language, to solve familiar problems, to think clearly, or to control feelings could be more devastating to the individual than the physical infirmities associated with stroke' (Levine and Zigler, 1975, p. 752). However, the evidence that patients with dysphasia are more depressed, for example, than other stroke patients, is not conclusive (Brocklehurst *et al.*, 1978*a*).

In the first weeks after stroke many patients must struggle to adjust to sudden changes in themselves and in their relationship to their environment. Assumed and unquestioned abilities may disappear – to drink a cup of tea, to visit the toilet alone; expectations of the future may be shattered and prospects for the future uncertain; the present may appear to contain only the humiliation of being fed and bathed and feelings of total dependence upon others. The term 'depression' is commonly used by patients, researchers and doctors to describe a variety of mood disorders following stroke. Different approaches to assessing the phenomenon of depression (Robinson and Price, 1982; Feibel and Springer, 1982; Wade, 1984) indicate that this is a common and persistent problem, affecting nearly one-third of patients over the first year after the stroke.

The longer-term outlook for many stroke survivors appears unpromising. Of patients discharged from an Australian hospital and followed-up 3 years later only one-quarter were optimistic about the future (Lawrence and Christie, 1979). In a 2–3-year follow-up study from Frenchay Hospital in Bristol, Holbrook (1982) reports that one-third of patients said they had not adjusted to the effects of the stroke, and many felt they never would. Isaacs and colleagues (1976) followed for 3 years 29 stroke patients who were discharged home. Although most remained physically fit, many became depressed and frustrated. Only 4 of these 29 survivors were described as adjusting successfully to the stroke; others had gone through changes in their personality towards aggression, frustration and a reluctance to co-operate or participate in normal living. One-quarter of the spouses of younger stroke survivors reported a marked personality change among patients discharged from a London rehabilitation centre (Coughlan and Humphrey, 1982); these included irritability, loss of self-control, impatience, lowered tolerance, frustration, emotional lability and reduced initiative. Spouses described life for 41% of patients as much less enjoyable than before the stroke, and 31% of the spouses said that they themselves now enjoyed life much less.

The impact of stroke on social and family life has been relatively neglected. Yet various studies (Hyman, 1971; Folstein *et al.*, 1977) suggest that the social reintegration of stroke patients is possibly the most problematic aspect of rehabilitation.

Survivors may become socially isolated not only because they lack the opportunity or inclination to visit friends or travel to social events, but also because there is a lack of appropriate facilities, such as day centres and restaurants, which are able to accommodate disabled people, and because old friends, colleagues and social contacts do not visit (Isaacs *et al.*, 1976). The stroke survivor may be a changed person, difficult to communicate with, distressing to meet, and with whom it seems embarrassing to discuss past occasions or future plans. Many patients will acquire the status of 'disabled', which is likely to attract a multitude of negative evaluations, extending into different spheres of life including work (Seifert, 1979).

Although less than a quarter of stroke victims are people of working age, this group survives better than older patients; thus, for example, in the sample of Weddell and Beresford (1979) one-third of the males alive at 3 months after stroke were of working age. Of the males in this study who had previously been employed full-time less than one-third had returned to full employment 3 months after the stroke. (In all age groups, nearly half the housewives said that they were working at the same level as before by 3 months after the stroke.)

The loss of employment may mean a reduction in income and financial difficulties for many patients, at a time when additional money may be necessary to cover new transport or housing costs, and when the ability to buy aids and appliances may be useful. M. Smith and colleagues (1981) note that extra expense was incurred by patients who bought aids for themselves, either because they found they needed them urgently, did not want to join a waiting list, or were unaware that aids could be obtained on loan.

A quarter of the younger (work-age) patients in the study of Mackay and Nias (1979) felt they had sustained a financial loss because of the stroke; and this figure is likely to be an underestimate for problems over the course of a year since interviews were held about 6 months after the stroke, and, in England, the obligation of employers to pay employees on sick leave ends after 6 months. Blaxter (1976), in a general study of physically disabled people, found that 'financial problems were likely to begin some 6 or 7 months after the illness episode'. A study of members of a stroke club in Seattle, at least 1 year after being discharged from a hospital treatment programme (Belcher *et al.*, 1978), revealed that the mean income of single stroke survivors was only one-third of the mean income for married stroke survivors. None of the single people were working, but 7% of the married stroke patients and 38% of their spouses were working. Clearly, single people recovering from stroke are less likely to have readily available support of many types than are their married counterparts. The financial consequences of stroke should be considered with regard to the entire household unit and not only the stroke patient.

Carers: their contribution and some consequences for their lives

Stroke is a 'family' illness; it presents challenges and dilemmas to those who live with or support patients. For stroke patients, and the chronically ill generally, the family is the main source of emotional, social and practical support (Henwood 1990). Since most stroke patients are elderly, it is important to establish their expectations about who should help when they are ill. Shanas (1979) reports that: 'Old people turn first to their families for help, then to neighbours, and finally, to the bureaucratic replacements for families – social workers, ministers, community agencies, and others – because they expect families to help in the case of need' (p. 174).

Changes in the attitudes and preferences of disabled people for different sources of support have received little attention; much more has been made of demographic changes – such as the growing numbers of dependent older people, rising rates of divorce, and the increasing proportion of women employed outside the home – and statements about the increasing reluctance of family members to care, as indications of an impending decline in the availability of family support. Firm evidence about changes in attitudes to caring is lacking, nor has a reduction in support given by the family been adequately documented (Allen *et al.*, 1987). In the Farnham study (Weddell and Beresford, 1979) nine-tenths of patients living with others at home 3 months after the stroke were receiving help from someone in the household; a quarter of all the survivors were being helped by members of the extended family. Among 67 survivors 4 years after the stroke, 9 received no help at all (either from their own families or anyone else), 45 had help in one or more ways from members of their own households, 7 had help from neighbours, and 14 from their extended family. There has clearly been growing awareness, if not appropriate recognition (Anderson, 1987), of the non-professional caring resource of family, neighbours, mutual aid and voluntary organisations. Both government and service providers acknowledge that family carers constitute the backbone of caring in the community, but they may be hesitant or uncertain about how to support the carers effectively (Twigg *et al.*, 1990). Many of the general needs of carers are well known (Anderson, 1987), but response to these needs will not be helped by the growing constraints on public expenditure, nor by long-established problems of co-ordinating care (Royal College of Physicians, 1986). A major focus of the chapters which follow will be the care given to stroke patients by family and friends, the difficulties that these carers experience, and the support that they receive from health and social services.

The reactions of the family and main supporters to the patient and to the stroke have been identified as significant influences on the patient's response to the stroke (Andrews, 1978) and to rehabilitation (Hyman, 1972), and on the patient's rate of progress towards recovery (Robertson and Suinn, 1968). The willingness and ability of the family to respond to, or organise a response to, problems of mobility, communication, money or other aspects of life may largely determine the likelihood of the patient remaining in a non-institutional environment (Sandford, 1975; Mykyta *et al.*, 1976). When the patient is living at home, the supporters appear to have an important role in determining use of, and satisfaction with services (Morrissey *et al.*, 1981; Field *et al.*, 1983); they also influence the amount that patients do for themselves and their subsequent progress in rehabilitation (Andrews and Stewart, 1979; Garraway *et al.*, 1980*a*).

Differences of opinion between the patient and family about what the patient can do (see New *et al.*, 1968) may lead either to 'overprotectiveness' or to the failure to give support when the stroke survivor needs it. Family members may feel anger and resentment towards the patient, though this may not always cause rejection; D'Afflitti and Weitz (1977) refer to families feeling guilt and resentment which was translated into overprotection of the patient. In a study of 79 stroke patients and their spouses Kinsella and Duffy (1979) reported that overprotection and unrealistic expectations among the spouses were a more common response than either rejection of the patient or retributive guilt feelings.

Relatives, mainly close family, are the main source of help and support for stroke patients, but they pay some price for this. A high proportion of people who support the survivors of a stroke identify deleterious effects of caring on their health and emotional well-being (Brocklehurst *et al.*, 1981). Depression among carers has been related to the patient's physical disability in some studies, but not others. However, the Frenchay study (Wade *et al.*, 1986*a*) indicates that, at least in the first year after the stroke, the carer's depression is related to the patient's emotional condition. Changes in the patient's mood or personality are often referred to, but their frequency among patients and their serious effects on the lives of supporters have been documented only for a sample of younger stroke survivors (Coughlan and Humphrey, 1982). Isaacs and colleagues (1976) point out that increased dependency upon contacts with close family and relatives may contribute to increasing conflict and hostility at home. This deterioration in family, particularly marital, relationships has been documented for dysphasic patients (Malone *et al.*, 1979) but not systematically for a complete series of stroke patients. The loss of the patient as an active social partner and the demands of patients which reduce the time or energy available for social activities may be an important cause of problems and distress for the patient's supporters. Among the spouses of younger stroke patients, the loss of companionship and interference with social and leisure activities were described as the major reasons for a loss of enjoyment of life (Coughlan and Humphrey, 1982). However, among the chief carers of patients in South Manchester, it is reported that the disruption of their leisure activities, which had been a significant feature shortly after the stroke, was minimal by the end of 1 year (Brocklehurst *et al.*, 1978*a*). The process of adjustment to a stroke is likely to vary with the age and relationship of the supporter to the patient, and certain issues are likely to be more salient at different stages after stroke, but there is little evidence as to how this pattern changes over time.

It is not known which of the various problems that supporters face cause them most distress; and increasing awareness of the family burden of stroke has produced little research to indicate why some families cope better or worse than others. Nevertheless, therapists, doctors and pyschologists in the United States and Europe have set up programmes encouraging relatives to join in mutual aid groups; to open communication between patient and family; to make more effective use of community medical and social services; and to increase the family's understanding of stroke and its consequences (Mykyta *et al.*, 1976; D'Afflitti and Weitz, 1977; Dzau and Boehme, 1978). These initiatives are dotted about the country, basically in pockets of local interest. There appears to be no coherent policy for the support of the carers of stroke patients.

Much of the variation in stroke care appears to depend upon a belief or otherwise that any therapy or intervention improves the mobility, morale or quality of life of either patients or carers. Service providers find it difficult to decide which interventions are worth while, in part because the welfare of stroke patients and their families has not been a major focus for interventions (unlike the patient's physical disability), and in part because relatively little is known about the experience, particularly in the longer term, of living with stroke. By investigating the everyday meanings of stroke, in terms of both consequences and significance, it is hoped to provide an assessment of needs that will be relevant to service providers, planners and policy makers.

CHAPTER TWO

The Greenwich stroke study

The aim of the Greenwich stroke study was to identify and follow the experiences of a population of stroke patients and their supporters, looking especially at the nature of their problems and at how they were helped to cope with these problems. The study is, therefore, intended to increase understanding about both the quality of support and the quality of life of stroke patients and their carers.

Greenwich health district in London was identified as a suitable area for the study for several reasons: the boundaries of the health authority were coterminous with those of the local authority, thus making it possible to specify the statutory services available in the area; services included a specialised stroke unit, as well as support groups for both patients and carers; it was estimated that the district's population of about 216 000 would generate an adequate number of stroke patients during the course of the study; and, most importantly, several of the district's main service providers had expressed support for the research.

Greenwich forms a triangle to the south of the River Thames, the river running for 14 kilometres along its northern boundary. The triangle contains contrasting social conditions, ranging from areas of comfortable owner-occupied houses to pockets of high unemployment and overcrowding. At the time of the study the local authority was having its income from local tax reduced by the government for overspending, while the health authority's budget was being reduced relative to other health districts because it was more than 20% overfunded in relation to the targets of the Resource Allocation Working Party. The health district has two main hospitals, both with accident and emergency units, rehabilitation departments and a day hospital: Greenwich District Hospital, which also has a specialist stroke unit with 24 beds; and the Brook General Hospital, which also houses specialist regional units for, among other things, neurosurgery, neurology and thoracic surgery. There were two smaller hospitals, with physiotherapy services, to which older patients were admitted – the Dreadnought Seaman's Hospital and St Nicholas' Hospital – but both have now closed. There is also one 96-bed, long-stay hospital to which some patients were transferred during the study.

General practice in Greenwich differs in some characteristics from the overall pattern in England. During the course of the study nearly 10% of the general practitioners retired or left the area, to be replaced by younger doctors. Information was provided by the Family Practitioner Committee on principals registered with them in early 1984 (about mid-way through the fieldwork on the study). Compared with figures on principals in England in 1983 (DHSS, 1985) Greenwich had a higher proportion of doctors working on their own rather than in a group practice (27% compared with 13% nationally) and more women doctors (34% compared with 20%). Also, while 23% of doctors in England had been born outside the UK or Ireland, 42% of doctors in Greenwich had qualified outside the UK or Ireland. Altogether 15% of doctors in Greenwich were aged 60 or more, which was just a little higher than the national average. These were the people – doctors in general practice and in hospital – whose support was necessary in order to identify people having strokes. There are obviously no convenient lists of people surviving to 3 weeks after a stroke; generating a study population of survivors meant developing a community register.

Identification of stroke patients

The register of strokes on which the study was based was intended to include all people aged 60 or over, registered with a general practitioner in Greenwich, who between April and December 1983 survived to at least 3 weeks after a stroke. There were no reasons for restricting the study population only to those receiving rehabilitation or with hemiplegia or who were treated in hospital. The only narrowing of interest was a decision to concentrate on patients aged 60 or over, who constitute five-sixths of all stroke patients. This is a group which has been relatively neglected in other studies and it was considered both more practical and more effective to focus in detail on these patients' needs and experiences. (As it turned out it would have been quite straightforward to have included younger patients, but some of their concerns – for example, being a parent of dependent children or a worker – were barely covered in the study.)

The adequacy of the stroke register depended upon the completeness of notifications of the diagnosis of stroke. The identification of people with a diagnosis of stroke raised ethical questions, including confidentiality, and led to the need for written support from individual doctors in the health district. All the consultants who were likely to have patients with stroke on their wards (21 of them) agreed in principle that patients under their care would be identified for the study. Altogether, after three mailings, 54% of the 124 general practitioners agreed to participate, 8% refused and 38% never replied. Doctors in 15 practices identified practice secretaries or receptionists as the key contacts.

Several systems were developed for notification of new stroke patients. The information required was, first, a diagnosis of stroke and the date of onset, based upon the report of the doctor. For patients alive at the time of examination, results from the WHO collaborative trial showed that stroke could be diagnosed accurately (Aho *et al.*, 1980), and in our study the doctors had up to 3 weeks after the stroke to revise their initial diagnosis. This was the only medical information required about the patients, and was given on the understanding that the researcher would neither inform nor confirm to patients that their diagnosis was stroke. The study was to be described to patients as investigating recovery from 'illness'. The only other information sought was name, address, date of birth (to check that the patient was aged 60 or over), and name of the patient's general practitioner (to check that the patient was registered with a doctor in Greenwich health district).

There were generally two parts to the notification, the first identifying the patient and the second giving the doctor's consent to approach the patient to seek participation in the study. Both parts were in most cases completed by the doctor, but on the general medical wards of one of the main hospitals it was agreed that patients would only be eligible for the study if they, or their next of kin, gave written informed consent for their diagnosis to be passed to the researcher. This system of notification was cumbersome since only a doctor could approach the patient to ask for their consent; as the junior doctors rotated between wards, new doctors had constantly to be informed of the system. All the medical, geriatric, orthopaedic and some of the surgical wards were visited every week to collect completed forms, and often to have forms signed. Altogether during the period from April to December 1983, 176 patients were identified who satisfied the criteria for inclusion in the study.

Some of the eligible stroke survivors are likely to have been 'missed' simply because only 54% of general practitioners in the health district confirmed their participation in the study. However, in London perhaps more so than in other urban areas of England (Brocklehurst *et al.*, 1978*b*; Wade and Langton-Hewer, 1985), relatively few patients are cared for exclusively by the general practitioner at home. A crude estimate of the completeness of the sample can be made using epidemiological data from other community registers. Since this is not a study of incidence, but essentially of survivors, the results from four studies in southern England (Weddell and Beresford, 1979; Stevens and Ambler, 1982; OCSP, 1983; Wade *et al.*, 1985*a*) have been aggregated to give rough estimates of incidence (2 per 1000), proportion of patients aged 60 or over (85%), and survival to 3 weeks (65%). Altogether, in a health district with a population the size of Greenwich (216 000) about 180 survivors could have been expected over the duration of the research; there were 176 in the study. However, none of the other studies were based in London and it seems reasonable to conclude that there is some shortfall in registration of strokes, largely due to a failure to identify a small number of milder cases managed at home.

The interviews

A major problem in this study of attitudes and experiences was identifying questions which were not only relevant and sensitive to the problems and changes in circumstances following stroke, but which also allowed for participation or response by the maximum proportion of patients. An attempt was made to screen patients for hearing (and usually to find their hearing aid), for comprehension and for orientation (the questions are in the Appendix). Patients were asked for their consent to the researcher checking some details with nursing and rehabilitation staff. It was decided to place a series of short clinical assessments immediately after this initial screening section (see Appendix) as both a further check on patients' ability to understand the interviewer, and an evaluation of the assessments' usefulness as predictors of recovery (Wade *et al.*, 1983).

The investigation of quality of life after stroke was considered in terms of both the conditions of life and the subjective evaluations of these conditions. Thus the questionnaires included measures of resources (employment, housing, money) and satisfaction with aspects of life (health, home, relationships). The Nottingham Health Profile (Hunt *et al.*, 1984), which demands only 'yes' or 'no' responses, was used to measure subjective aspects of well-being. (The study instruments are described in the Appendix.)

In any study, but particularly a longitudinal survey, it is important to maintain the trust and confidence of respondents. In this study, people were being asked about their personal response to illness and about their feelings towards people around them. There could be no question of information from or about one person being passed on to someone else, so it was decided that patients and their supporters should be interviewed separately. (All patients were seen by the author. The researcher who saw all the supporters had no information about the patient other than name and relationship to the supporter.)

In order to document the pattern of recovery, phases of emotional response to the stroke and points of crisis or difficulty, patients and supporters were interviewed three times in the 18 months after the stroke. The first interview was not sought until after the early phase of high mortality. On the basis of previous studies a cohort of longer-term survivors should have emerged by about 3 weeks after the stroke. An initial interview was conducted then to document impairment, disability and use of acute services, and, as far as possible, to establish the details of everyday life before the stroke. The timing of this interview is comparable with that in several other studies of stroke patients (Brocklehurst *et al.*, 1978*a*; Weddell and Beresford, 1979; Wade *et al.*, 1983; Warlow *et al.*, 1987). It was planned that patients should be seen again about 6 months later to report on their experiences of, and attitudes to, care and rehabilitation. This would also be a time when, for many, physical recovery had slowed down, but when there are many social and economic difficulties (Blaxter, 1976; Holbrook, 1982). Final contact would be made a further 8–9 months later when physical recovery had probably peaked. Outcome *at that stage* would be assessed in terms of disability and morbidity, but also considering changes in domestic and social activities, subjective assessments of health, recovery, quality of life and attitudes to the future.

The study reviews a particular segment of time in the lives of these patients and their supporters. At different stages of the study the interviews concentrated upon experiences and statuses in different areas of life. However, the cornerstone of the attempt to assess the consequences of the stroke was the documentation of changes in everyday life since the illness – in mobility and self-care, leisure and household activities, family and social relationships, and in subjective health. These dimensions of outcome pertained also to the assessment of consequences for the supporters, but additionally the study focused upon changes in the supporter's views of the patient, the patient's personality and their relationship.

Response to interviews

Altogether 98% of patients were assessed. Only 3 patients refused to participate: 2 did not want their diagnosis passed on to the researcher, and 1 decided after some consideration that he did not wish to participate, believing his diagnosis was psychiatric rather than stroke. Ultimately he declined to participate because he doubted assurances about the confidentiality of any information he gave. This patient was not unusual in being unaware of his main diagnosis (at the first interview only 63% of those who were able to respond to a question about what was wrong with them mentioned stroke, 10% reported some other health problem, and 27% said they did not know what was wrong); it was both a paradox and dilemma not to be able to 'reassure' the patient that it was 'only' a stroke.

It was intended that for each patient a supporter should be identified as 'the person who, in general, gives you most help and support'. This was not necessarily, therefore, someone who gave practical help, but someone who could be providing support by visiting, giving information, showing concern, helping to sort out problems, or improving the patient's morale. If the patient was unable to communicate for any reason then the identification of the main supporter was sought from the patient's family or a ward nurse. Altogether main supporters were identified for 160 of the patients: in 6 cases no one appeared to act as a supporter for the patient, and in 7 cases the patient refused to pass on the name of the main supporter. Patients were reassured about the confidentiality of the supporter's interviews and told that they would be conducted by another interviewer who knew nothing about the patients; but the patients' main objection was to having their supporters 'bothered' when they were already worried or burdened enough.

In Chapter 5, the survival of patients will be discussed in detail. However, it is apparent in this study that the wave of high mortality following the stroke was not over by the end of the first month. Many patients were still very unwell when first seen, and 11 died in the next few days before their main supporter was visited. One supporter also died in the days between the patients' and supporters' interview. So, altogether 148 supporters were available for a first interview. The response rates at the first and subsequent interviews are shown in Table 1.

The term 'interview' is a generous description for some of the contacts: at the first interview 19 patients were too ill to provide more than a few items of information; at the second interview 3 patients were too ill: and at the third interview 2 patients were too ill. However, the interviews combined questions about everyday life (housing, walking, shopping,

Table 1. *The response rates of patients and supporters*

	Patients' interview			Supporters' interview		
	1st	2nd	3rd	1st	2nd	3rd
Eligible	176	116	96	148	101	80
Interviewed	173	110	93	147	95	76
Response rate	98%	95%	97%	99%	94%	95%
No. of deaths before next phase (patients + 1 supporter)	57	14		46	15	

going to the pub, using services) and questions about attitudes (to recovery, services, spouse). Information about the former activities was also drawn from interviews with supporters and nurses when the patient was too ill, confused or speech-impaired to represent himself or herself.*

The interviews with the patients, and shortly afterwards with their supporters, took place at around 4 weeks (T1), 9 months (T2) and 18 months (T3) after the stroke (88% were seen between the third and fifth weeks; 96% between the eighth and tenth month after the stroke). Excluding contacts when the patient was too ill for a useful interview, the interviews lasted, on average, about 1 hour each, although they were somewhat shorter than this for a majority of patients at their first interview, and significantly longer for most supporters at their first interview. The distribution of the duration of the interviews is in Table 2.

The patients

The patients are a cohort of *survivors* from stroke – of people aged 60 and over who lived beyond the acute phase of 3 weeks after a stroke. As would be expected from the epidemiological data, there was a small majority of women (55%) and a higher proportion of people aged 75 or over (58%).

---

* One of the main difficulties in this study was to obtain complete and valid information on activities from or for patients with speech impairments, mental confusion or other difficulties in communication. All patients were interviewed by the same person (R.A.) who recorded observations of their performance at the time of interviewing. Information on the same questions was obtained from the patient's supporter and where appropriate, from nursing staff. The use of information from different sources has problems but, together with personal observations, has been used to make 'best' judgements about the patient's performance of daily activities.

Table 2. *Duration of interviews*

	Patients'			Supporters'		
Duration of interview	1st (%)	2nd (%)	3rd (%)	1st (%)	2nd (%)	3rd (%)
Less than 40 minutes	18	16	18	1	11	17
40–59 mintues	40	31	37	23	41	33
60–79 minutes	30	30	29	45	29	36
80 minutes or longer	12	23	16	31	19	14
No. of interviews (= 100%)	154	107	89	146	94	76

The age and sex of patients were related: 19% of men were aged 80 or over compared with 38% of women.* Associated with this age difference, 65% of women were widowed and 21% married, compared with 29% of men who were widowed and 59% who were married at the time of stroke.

The patients all came from one part of London; their lives and experiences should not be considered typical of elderly people elsewhere in Great Britain, though in many respects, as will be noted, they are similar (cf. OPCS, 1982). One marked difference from the national pattern was their housing before the stroke: relatively few (24%) lived in their own homes, while a high proportion (55%) were in the public sector (council houses, sheltered housing and residential homes for the elderly). The proportion of people living in sheltered housing or a residential home increased from 9% of people aged 60–69, to 13% of those aged 70–79, and up to 27% of patients aged 80 or over.

At the time of the stroke nearly half the patients were living on their own, compared with a third of elderly people in Great Britain as a whole (OPCS, 1982); this proportion increased with age and was higher for women in all age groups. The figures are given in Table 3.

Only 20% of women lived with their spouse compared with 56% of men. Altogether 18% of the stroke patients were living with children; but 80% had living children (30% had one child, 24% two children, 12% three children, 7% four children, and 7% five children or more).

Most of the patients had experienced what could be described as fairly hard lives, typically working in the local armaments factory, or in trades associated with the River Thames. Only 14 people were in paid employ-

* Unless otherwise stated, attention has not been drawn to differences which might have occurred by chance 5 or more times in 100.

Table 3. *Proportions of patients living alone before the stroke, by age and sex*

Age	Men		Women		All	
60–69	11%	(18)[a]	35%	(17)	23%	(35)
70–79	23%	(43)	61%	(41)	42%	(84)
80+	43%	(14)	79%	(33)	68%	(47)
All	24%	(75)	63%	(91)	45%	(166)

[a] Figures in brackets are the numbers upon which percentages are based (= 100%).

ment at the time of the stroke; 5 of these were part-time. It is often difficult to classify the social class of these older people because they have done different jobs during working lives interrupted by two world wars. A large majority (83%) left school at the earliest possible age, often to go into factory work or, in the case of women, into domestic service. Occasionally patients, particularly widows, had trouble identifying their, or their husbands', occupation, but this was usually a problem with defining the nature of different unskilled labouring jobs. It was possible to classify the social class of 84% of the patients on the basis of their main occupation during their working lives. Married and widowed women were classified by their husband's occupation, which may be a less dubious exercise among older populations in which few of the women have had long-term, full-time employment. Nevertheless, it has been suggested that housing tenure may be a better indicator of social values and lifestyle than is occupation-based social class. As can be seen in Table 4, for this group social class and tenure were related.

Altogether, two-thirds of patients were in owner-occupied or council housing; it is clear how these categories of tenure relate to ideas of social class, but difficult to see how the social class of the remaining third of patients should be analysed. Moreover, housing type may be changed by the onset of disability and is one of the outcome variables in this study. For these reasons, careful questioning was used to classify patients by social class rather than housing tenure.

Most of the patients were in reasonable health and independent in activities of daily living before the stroke. Altogether 35% of patients rated their health for their age as excellent before the stroke, 39% as good, 23% as fair and 3% as poor. These subjective assessments are relatively positive compared with random samples of the elderly population

Table 4. *Social class and housing tenure of patients*

Tenure	Social class				
	I + II: professional and intermediate (%)	III: non-manual (%)	III: skilled manual (%)	IV + V: semi-skilled and unskilled (%)	All patients (%)
Owner occupier	50	43	22	13	24
Council housing	14	22	40	55	40
Private rented	14	14	12	7	10
Sheltered + residential homes	4	14	15	16	16
Home of family /friends	18	7	11	9	10
No. of patients (= 100%)[a]	22	14	65	45	158

[a]In this and other tables small numbers of patients on whom inadequate information was obtained on particular questions have been omitted.

(OPCS, 1982; Cartwright and Smith, 1988). Among the patients women more often viewed their health for their age as having been only fair or poor – 35% described it like this compared with 16% of men. The differences between men and women were largely among patients aged 60–79; 44% of women in this age group described their health as fair or poor, but only 17% of men said this.

Self-rating of health for age was associated with reporting the existence of a long-standing illness or disability; altogether 60% of patients said they were troubled by a long-standing illness, and 39% of those with a long-standing illness rated their health for their age as fair or poor, compared with 11% of those who did not mention a chronic illness. The most common illnesses that patients mentioned were, in order of frequency, rheumatism and arthritis (identified by 24% of those who said they had a chronic illness), cardiac problems and angina (16%), bronchial or lung diseases (13%) and high blood pressure (11%). When a specific enquiry was made to establish whether the patient had previously experienced a stroke, 36% answered that they had, which is a higher proportion than in other recent studies (cf. Brocklehurst *et al.*, 1978a; OCSP, 1983).

The proportion of patients who reported a long-standing illness or disability was not associated with the patient's sex, and although the proportion appeared to increase with age – from 48% of people in their

Table 5. *Age, sex and disability before the stroke*

	Proportion with little or no physical disability					
Age	Men		Women		All	
60–69	94%	(18)[a]	88%	(17)	91%	(35)
70–79	88%	(42)	72%	(39)	80%	(81)
80 +	71%	(14)	53%	(32)	59%	(46)
All aged 60 +	86%	(74)	68%	(88)	77%	(162)

[a] Figures in brackets are the numbers on which percentages are based (= 100%).

sixties, to 59% of those in their seventies, to 68% of people aged 80 or over – this trend was not statistically significant. Not surprisingly, people reporting a long-term illness were more physically disabled before the stroke: only 69% had little or no disability, compared with 91% of those without a chronic illness.

In the general population social class is related to reporting of chronic illness and disability, although the pattern is less marked among people aged 65 and over (OPCS, 1982). In this cohort of stroke survivors there was no association between level of disability before the stroke and social class, but, as expected, disability levels before the onset of this stroke were related to age and sex. Altogether, 77% of patients scored 15 or 16 for pre-stroke disability, based upon questions about activities of daily living (for details on scoring see Appendix) – which means little or no problem with mobility or self-care. But the proportion scoring 15 or 16 was higher among men and younger patients. The figures are given in Table 5.

Before the stroke, 25% of patients needed some help to walk outdoors, and women were more likely to need help than men (37% compared with only 11% of men). Many patients were reported to be receiving some help with looking after themselves before the stroke, and again the proportion was higher for women patients (63%) than for men (42%). However, these high figures are principally for help from a chiropodist with cutting toenails.

The patient's level of disability was related to the performance of activities, both domestic and social. Among patients with little or no disability, 94% were doing some housework (cooking, washing dishes, washing clothes, cleaning, shopping) compared with only 53% of those who scored 14 or less on the disability index. However, among those with little or no disability, men were doing less housework than women; for example, only 25% of men prepared a meal most days compared with 65%

Table 6. *Participation by patients in social activities over the 3 months before the stroke*

Frequency of participation	Social activities						
	Visit family/ friends (%)	Go to church (%)	Go to social club (%)	Go to pub (%)	Go on a day trip (%)	Go to an event (%)	Someone visits (%)
Never	37	90	75	80	65	91	5
1–2 times	15	1	2	4	19	4	7
3–12 times	14	3	4	3	14	4	18
Weekly +	34	6	19	13	2	1	70
No. of patients (=100%)	161	161	160	161	160	160	159

of women. Altogether, only 12% of patients were managing their housework without any help. Clearly those patients who were doing less received more help; supporters reported that 79% of male patients were receiving help from them with housework compared with 54% of female patients.

The social activities of patients were mainly oriented to contacts with family and friends. Few of the patients went out to a club, pub or entertainment on a regular basis. Their social activities in the 3 months before the stroke are described in Table 6.

The summary activities score for these patients averaged 13.0 (for scoring see Appendix). This score was higher for patients with little or no pre-stroke disability: they scored an average of 13.6 compared with 10.9 for patients with a disability score of 14 or less.

In summary, it appears that the homes and lives of most of the patients in the study were quite modest. There were many differences between men and women – from household to housework – associated in part with the high proportion of women among people aged 80 and over. Although other illnesses were common, the majority of patients were independent before the stroke in activities of daily living. However, they were a relatively home-oriented group whose social activities were principally contacts with family and friends. We next look at the lives of these contacts, who constitute the pool from which the main supporters have been drawn.

The supporters

The main carers of stroke patients have been identified in three of the recent British studies: in Manchester (Brocklehurst *et al.*, 1981), Edinburgh (Murray *et al.*, 1982) and Bristol (Wade *et al.*, 1986*a*). There are some differences between the studies in their definition of a carer; in particular the Bristol study included only people who lived with the patient. This matters because in the other studies between one-sixth (Brocklehurst *et al.*, 1981) and one-third (Murray *et al.*, 1982) of the main carers did not live in the same household as the patient. The age of the patient and whether the carer lives in or outside the patient's household affect the nature of the relationship between patient and carer; older patients, for example, are less likely to have a living spouse. In Manchester, three-fifths of the carers were spouses; in Edinburgh the proportion was slightly less than half; in Greenwich it was just over one-third.

Among patients aged 60–79, 46% of supporters were spouses and 35% were children (an inappropriate label perhaps, considering that no supporter was aged under 25); among patients aged 80 or over only 5% of the main supporters were spouses, and 67% were sons or daughters (including in-laws). Altogether, just over a third of the supporters were aged 65 or over.

There was no significant difference in the sex of supporters in different age groups. Most supporters (65%) were caring for a patient of the opposite sex; in just over half of these cases the supporter was the patient's spouse. The relationships of the supporters to the patients are shown in Table 7. If spouses are excluded from consideration, then 33% of women patients were receiving their main support from a man (usually their son), and 76% of men had a female supporter. At the time of the stroke half of the supporters were living with the patient, including all spouses and 28% of sons and daughters. Male and female supporters were equally likely to be sharing their home with the patient but the proportion of supporters doing this increased with age, from 23% of those aged under 40 to 79% of those aged 65 and over.

Altogether, 88% of the supporters were relatives of the stroke patient. Thus the proportion drawn from family is very high, as in the other stroke studies (Brocklehurst *et al.*, 1981; Murray *et al.* 1982), even though the patients in Greenwich were relatively old and the proportion of supporters who lived with the patient was comparatively low. Most relationships were long-standing, so that nearly 90% of these patients and supporters had known each other for 20 years or longer.

Among patients who were married, 89% of the carers were their

Table 7. *The relationships of supporters to patients, by sex of patients*

Relationship of the supporter	Sex of patient		All supporters (%)
	Male (%)	Female (%)	
Wife	52	0	24
Husband	0	19	10
Daughter(-in-law)	15	38	27
Son(-in-law)	12	22	17
Sister	7	5	6
Brother	0	1	1
Other relative	4	3	3
Friend	7	6	7
Other 'carer'	3	6	5
No. of patients (= 100%)	68	79	147

spouses; the spouse was not identified as the main supporter when they themselves were ill (and usually the patient had been supporting them), or when someone else in the household usually gave more support or was seen by the patient as fitter and more likely to give most help in the future. When the patients were widowed, divorced or separated 77% of the supporters were sons or daughters; that is, 86% of this group who had been married and who had living children identified a child as the main supporter. If the patient was widowed, divorced or separated and had any daughters, then a daughter was identified as the main supporter in 71% of cases; if, in the same circumstances the patient had any sons, then a son was identified in 48% of cases. Daughters, then, were more often identified as supporters than were sons.

All the supporters in the categories of 'other' relatives and 'carers' (four home helps, two care assistants and a social worker) were women; altogether 70% of the main supporters were women. So, in this study as in others, most of the burden of caring falls on women (Anderson, 1987). Nevertheless, the presence of men as carers is substantial; carers are a heterogenous group and there is a need for caution in the use of simple stereotypes.

The supporters expressed a rather negative view of their health; at the first interview only 12% of supporters rated their health for their age as excellent, 50% described it as good, but 38% said it was only fair or poor. This last figure is higher than the proportion of patients (26%) who rated their health for their age as fair or poor. The supporter's subjective assessment of his or her health was poorer if, before the stroke, the patient had been disabled: the proportion rating their health for their age as fair or poor was 33% among those supporting patients who had little or no disability, but 53% among those supporting patients with higher levels of physical disability before the stroke. In 15% of cases both patient and supporter rated their own health for their age as fair or poor.

Supporters' rating of health for their age was not, overall, related to their sex; but among those aged under 65 only 14% of men described their health as fair or poor compared with 39% of women.

As would be expected, supporters who rated their health less positively were much more likely to say they suffered with some long-standing illness or disability: 85% of those rating their health as fair or poor identified some such problem, but only 40% of those who described their health as excellent or good. Altogether, 58% of the supporters mentioned a chronic health problem. These problems were similar to those identified by the patients; the most common were, in order of frequency, rheumatism and arthritis, cardiac problems, chest and bronchial complaints and high blood pressure. None of the patients mentioned any problems with nerves, but nearly 1 in 10 of the supporters volunteered that they had a problem with depression or headaches. Among supporters 65% of women identified a long-standing health problem, compared with 41% of men. There was a consistent increase with age in the proportion who reported a chronic illness, rising from 29% of the supporters under age 45 up to 84% of those aged 75 and over.

Altogether, 79% of supporters were currently married, 6% single, 10% widowed and 5% divorced or separated. All the widowed were women. Eighty-two per cent of supporters had some living children and, at the time of the stroke, a quarter of the supporters were living with children at home. Nearly half of the supporters lived with their spouse only, and 1 in 15 lived alone. Half of these supporters were a generation younger than the patients; not surprisingly, then, more of the supporters (53%) lived in owner-occupied homes. Another 33% were in council property, 9% in privately rented accommodation, and 5% lived with family or in other arrangements.

Nearly half (48%) of the supporters were in paid employment before the stroke but, not surprisingly, this figure comprised 72% of carers aged under 65 and only 6% of people aged 65 and over. Among the main group of employed people, aged 25 to 64, men were both more likely to be employed and to work longer hours. The figures are given in Table 8.

There were no age or sex differences in the proportions of supporters who, before the patient's stroke, had commitments to and spent time on

Table 8. *Paid employment of supporters,[a] by sex*

	Supporters		
No. of hours worked weekly before the stroke	Men (%)	Women (%)	All (%)
None	7	38	28
Less than 20	0	11	7
20–29	7	14	12
30–39	31	28	29
40 or more	55	9	24
No. of supporters (= 100%)	29	64	93

[a] Only supporters aged 25–64 are considered.

Table 9. *Participation by supporters in social activities over the 3 months before the stroke*

	Social activities							
Frequency of participation (%)	Visit family (%)	Go to church (%)	Go to social club (%)	Go to pub (%)	Go on a day trip (%)	Go to a sports event (%)	Visit theatre, cinema (%)	Someone visits (%)
Never	12	86	72	70	57	85	77	6
1–2 times	8	5	2	3	19	5	10	8
3–12 times	17	2	7	11	22	3	12	18
Weekly +	63	7	19	16	2	7	1	68
No. of supporters (= 100%)	145	145	145	145	145	145	145	145

voluntary work. Seventeen per cent of supporters said they did this; their activities ranged from hospital visiting and church activities to participation in the women's fellowship, trade unions, tenants' associations and school governors' work. These organisations for voluntary work were heavily represented in the lists of clubs and societies of which the supporters were members. Men were more likely to belong to a club or society; 56% of them did, compared with 29% of women. The former went to working men's clubs and workplace social clubs as well as sports clubs of various kinds. There was no sex difference in membership of a church or religious organisation, which stood at 13%

On the whole hobbies of the supporters were based at home, and the social activities of the supporters, like those of the patients, were dominated by visits to and from family and friends. The frequencies of different social activities in the 3 months before the patient's stroke are shown in Table 9.

The summary activities score for supporters' lives before the stroke averaged 15.9 (for scoring see Appendix); it was higher for people aged under 65 than for those aged 65 or over (16.4 compared with 14.9), and it was greater for men than for women (17.0 compared with 15.4). This sex difference was due to more frequent patronage of the pub by men (30% went at least once a week but only 10% of the women supporters) and because men more often went to sports and other events – 28% had been at least once in the 3 months before the stroke compared with 10% of women.

SUMMARY

This chapter presents details on the methods and subjects of the study in Greenwich. Information on the lives and health of the patients and supporters before the stroke provides a basis for assessing how, and for whom, the illness changed their lives. Subsequent chapters describe how the nature and quality of these lives were affected by the stroke and consider what contribution different factors, but especially health and social services, made to the process of change following stroke.

The research is based upon a community register of people surviving beyond the acute phase of stroke in Greenwich health district (which has boundaries coterminous with those of the local authority). There were three major difficulties in setting up the study: generating support from doctors and the various committees in the health district; developing a system for notification of new strokes; and designing a questionnaire that could be used with patients who had impaired communication. Patients and their carers often viewed the patient's activities from different perspectives, indicating a need for caution in the use of information from proxy respondents.

Altogether 173 eligible patients were entered into the study during 9 months from April to December 1983. These were all people aged 60 or over, registered with a general practitioner in Greenwich health district, who survived for at least 3 weeks following a stroke. This number of patients was close to the figure expected on the basis of other epidemiological studies. The patients were asked for the identity of the person who gave them most help and support, and for permission to contact this 'informal' supporter. Patients and their supporters (99% of whom agreed to participate) were interviewed separately by different people at 1, 9 and 18 months after the stroke.

The patients The patients are a cohort of survivors from stroke; however they reflect the pattern of incidence, with a small majority of women (55%) and a higher proportion of people aged 75 or over (58%). The age and sex of the patients were related: 19% of men were aged 80 or over compared with 38% of women. At the time of stroke nearly half the patients were living alone, and only 20% of women were living with their spouse compared with 56% of men. Three-quarters of the patients were classified as working-class, and more than half of all patients were living in public sector housing. Sixty per cent of patients said they had been troubled by a long-standing illness before the stroke, but only a quarter had any appreciable problem with mobility or self-care. A third of the patients had had a previous stroke. Disability levels before the onset of the stroke were related to age and sex; and 63% of women compared with 42% of men were receiving some help before the stroke (mainly with chiropody). The patient's level of disability was clearly related to the performance of activities, both domestic and social.

The supporters These were drawn overwhelmingly (88%) from the family of the stroke patient; altogether 70% of the carers were women. The supporters identified by patients were generally spouses, if alive, followed by children; among patients aged 80 or over only 5% of the main supporters were spouses, but 67% were children, mainly daughters. Altogether, half the supporters were living with the patient before the stroke. More than a third of the supporters were aged 65 or over, and half of these older supporters rated their health as only fair or poor. In general, the quality of the relationship between patients and supporters before the stroke was good, two-thirds rating it as 'very happy'. Before the stroke the supporters had a range of commitments: nearly half were in paid work, a quarter had children living at home, and most led fairly active social lives. Among both patients and supporters most social activities were centred around home, family and friends.

The following chapters take up the theme of how stroke changes the lives of patients and carers. Topics are dealt with essentially chrono-logically, starting with the onset of the illness, the entry of the patients into medical care, the early disability and how patients and carers coped with this.

CHAPTER THREE

Coming into medical care: the first month after stroke

The onset of the stroke

Following the onset of symptoms the patient or a carer must make decisions about whether to seek medical help and, if so, whether to contact the general practitioner or go direct to hospital. The typical scenario is thought to involve the sudden loss of movement or speech leading to rapid consultation with the general practitioner, who decides whether the patient should be cared for at home or referred to hospital. In general, this appears not to have been the experience of patients in Greenwich. Two points should be noted when comparing these patients with other series: first, since it is a study of survivors many of the patients with poor prognostic signs for survival of the stroke – for example, unconsciousness (Oxbury et al., 1975; Aho et al., 1980) – are excluded; secondly, no other study has been done in London, and in Greenwich no patient is more than 8 kilometres from a district general hospital.

At the time of onset of the stroke 83% of patients were at home, 6% were in, or attending, the hospital, and 11% were at work or elsewhere – a distribution similar to that in other studies of all strokes (e.g. Wade, 1984). However, it was apparent in the responses of patients and supporters to the question 'What happened?' that the definition of time of onset was often difficult. The majority of patients were not struck by a 'bolt from the blue' but usually found that suddenly they were unable to do something that they usually took for granted (making a cup of tea, talking on the phone, walking to the toilet) and then became engaged in a process of interpretation of the symptoms and attempts to control the emerging illness (see Alonzo, 1980). This often involved self-treatment and consultation with others. A widow in her mid-sixties, living alone at home, reported her experience:

I walked down this hill with no one to help me. I said to a woman [on the bus] 'My arm's a bit funny. I've got pins and needles.' When I got off the bus I couldn't see. I don't know how I did it ... I phoned my daughter and told her I felt ill. She naturally said to take two tablets and go to bed. I got up next morning worse than ever, phoned my daughter and said, crying, that I felt frightened. Tom, my son-in-law came. I was falling about here and Tom caught me three times. He said 'What's wrong Mum?' and I said 'I think I've had a little stroke.' 'Don't be silly' he said. But he rang my daughter and said 'Call the doctor'.

Other responses show how patients and their supporters waited for symptoms to develop before seeking help. The neighbour of a single woman living alone recalled:

I suspected it when she lost the use of the left side of her body. It happened on a Saturday. By the Tuesday the face had gone on one side and I knew there was something wrong and I phoned the doctor.

And the friend of a woman aged 77 told a similar story:

She was working in the garden and she came in and went to write and her hand slipped across the page and she had difficulty walking. The next day I found she couldn't spear her food. Then I took her to the doctor.

When patients collapse or are found unconscious the action of carers is generally to seek help immediately, but it appears that the symptoms of most strokes among survivors are less dramatic, even when they lead to severe disability, as it did in the following case, recounted by a semi-retired accountant:

The difficulty here is when did the illness begin. I walked across the grass verge and opened the garage door. As I walked across I felt a little giddy – I thought, 'What's wrong with me?' I came inside after getting the car out and sat down in this room to answer the phone. I picked it up, said 'Hello' and I suddenly noticed I was talking the most utter nonsense and gibberish. When my wife came home I was speaking the same as I am now, but worse, so my wife called Dr Meehan. I could walk then but when I came to go downstairs I couldn't get down all the way and had to sit on the stairs. When I got downstairs into the lounge I couldn't walk. You might say my stroke developed, rather than happened at one time. This was a shock to me because I thought the stroke came like the blinding flash to Paul on the road to Damascus. And I wish I'd known that 'cos if I had, when my speech became blurred I might have come upstairs and laid down and avoided some of the worst of the stroke.

Among the common reasons for delay in seeking medical help was the preference of patients to discuss their condition first with a friend or family member. If the symptoms began in the night it may not have been

convenient to call for help until morning, even if the patient was distressed. A widow who lived round the corner from her sister related her
discovery of the stroke:

As a matter of fact, I was just going to get out of bed to go to the toilet. When I
went to get up I couldn't get out of bed. I was struggling to get myself out of the
side. When finally I collected myself, I went to the kitchen but I couldn't make a
cup of tea or anything. I was really frightened by that. Later, when I thought my
sister was up, I phoned her and said 'I think I've had another stroke.'

Previous experience of stroke may be one factor influencing how
patients, and supporters, respond to symptoms, but it does not necessarily
imply urgency; awareness that the symptoms indicate a stroke may, as in
the following case of a widow living alone, provide an apparently satisfactory explanation which demands no particular response:

I was sitting by the fire eating when I couldn't get my food into my mouth. I went
to look in the mirror and saw the left side of my mouth was up. I knew it was a
stroke because my husband had one, but I didn't worry about it because I didn't
feel queer so I left it at that. On Sunday my daughter visited me here and said I
didn't look well. That upset me and I said I'd had a mild stroke. She said she knew
that so she and her husband took me to the hospital.

Of course, the mental processes, or coping strategies, by which people
attempt to control or come to terms with symptoms are complex. The
presence of 'denial' (Levine and Zigler, 1975), for example, is difficult to
chart. However, there were several instances in which patients asked the
supporters not to bother, or in which they sought to deny the significance
of the symptoms or to attribute the problem to something other than
stroke. The wife of a man in his early seventies reported that:

It took him a long time to understand he'd had a stroke. He couldn't understand
why he couldn't walk or stand. He went to do his part-time job. He was driving his
van – he stopped for the traffic, felt a bit groggy and went over. The girl in the car
behind came and knocked on his window. He said he had dozed off. Then he
carried on. He came home late – he dragged his leg a bit and said he thought he'd
pulled a muscle. Then he went upstairs for an hour. I phoned my daughter and
said 'You'd better come. I think he's had a stroke.' Then I phoned the doctor.

Seeking medical help

The decision to seek medical help in the case of stroke is, as with less
threatening illness, influenced by social factors and the local circumstances at the time of onset. There are so many possible factors and
courses of action that it is not possible to isolate different effects in a

general study such as this. However, it is evident that among the most important 'triggers' (Zola, 1973) to seeking medical care is consultation with and action of family and friends. In about one-fifth of the cases it appears that the decision was taken entirely by someone other than the patient – the patient having collapsed and been found unconscious.

Having decided that medical help should be sought the second decision about coming into medical care is whom to contact. On the basis of reports from patients and supporters the course of action was established for 153 of the 173 patients (most of the other 20 were too ill for interview and died before the supporter was interviewed). Nine patients were in hospital at the time of the stroke; of those living in the community 60% contacted a general practitioner and 40% went, or were taken direct, to hospital. This is clearly a high proportion going direct to hospital, compared with figures of 5% in Oxfordshire (Bamford *et al.*, 1986) 12% in Bristol (Wade and Langton-Hewer, 1985) and 22% in Manchester (Brocklehurst *et al.*, 1978b). However, the higher figure for Greenwich is compatible with other reports on the use of accident and emergency services in the capital (London Health Planning Consortium, 1981: The Acheson Report), and is lower than the proportion of strokes seen as direct emergency cases in a central London teaching hospital (A.-M. Tupper, personal communication).

The proportion of patients going directly to hospital was most clearly related to the patient's social class. The proportion increased consistently from 0% among patients from social classes 1 and 2, to 59% of patients from social class 5. The finding parallels that from a national study of use of services in an emergency: middle-class people are more likely to contact their own general practitioner (Cartwright and Anderson, 1981). It was suggested in the report of the national study that working-class patients may be less confident that the doctor will come out in an emergency, and some of the comments from patients and supporters in Greenwich identify this problem, but these unprompted comments cannot be analysed by social class.

The association between the decision about where to seek medical care and social class is difficult to explain. Only two other variables were associated with the decision and they are not related to social class. It appears that older patients may treat the onset differently: 89% of people aged 85 and over contacted their doctor compared with 55% of younger patients. Possibly the signs and symptoms are less threatening to old people because they are more common or expected. Among people with an existing chronic illness 69% contacted their general practitioner compared with 54% of the patients without a chronic illness, but the difference is not quite statistically significant. Patients with experience of a previous stroke were no more or less likely to contact their doctor. Nor were severity of the disability, side of stroke, or problems with comprehension or orientation related to the decision about whom to consult. The degree of speech impairment was an important factor: only 47% of the patients with loss of expression went to their general practitioner compared with 67% of patients who had no problem expressing themselves. This may be because patients with loss of speech are unable to telephone their doctor but know there will be care available at the hospital. It may be that speech loss is viewed as an unusual or a dramatic problem, but perception of severity of the stroke by patients and carers was not associated with the decision about where to seek help. Perhaps surprisingly the patient's household size, and whether he or she lived alone or was married, were not related to contacting the doctor, nor was sex of the patient.

The decision to go direct to hospital appeared to be more common when the patient was found unconscious, and also when the stroke occurred outside the patient's home (altogether 38% of patients who were at home at the time of the stroke went direct to hospital compared with 55% of patients who were elsewhere, but this difference was not statistically significant). A bachelor in his mid-seventies was going to lunch with his sister-in-law:

I got on the bus and when you get on those buses, he goes ding with the bell, through goes the clutch and you're through the window if you're not careful. I got up at New Cross, rang the bell. He jars and yanks this bloody bus and next minute I'm lying on the platform. Some men put me on the seat and the policeman came to ask me questions. It was a bit awkward then 'cos my speech was a bit slurred. He said he'd see my sister-in-law and try not to fear her. Then the ambulance man came and brought me in here. I've no idea what caused it. I considered myself to be in good shape before this.

Similarly, a stroke, recognised as such, which occurs in the middle of the night, when it is perhaps expected that the general practitioner is not available, may be likely to result in an emergency call. A woman who lived in sheltered housing with her husband reported that:

He's been under the doctor for years for high blood pressure. He said one day he had a funny headache – he went to bed, woke up and wanted to go to the bathroom. His legs were all funny. We sent for the warden at 3 a.m. He rang for the ambulance and they took him away. You could guess it was a stroke. It was all down one side and he couldn't speak properly. I guessed because he had one 3 years ago.

Several of the comments made by patients and supporters indicated that the decision to go straight to hospital was a reflection of the current or past response from their general practitioner. A man in his mid-seventies, living alone, had a sister who popped in every day to see him; she recalled:

He was half paralysed down one side. A couple of months ago he was ill. He thought he'd got 'flu – we thought he'd had a stroke. We sent for the doctor but his own doctor was away. I wrote to his own doctor saying we were worried about him – the doctor wrote a prescription but didn't go back. One day he was very ill. We sent for an ambulance – he's been in the Brook since then.

And a man who shared a flat with his sister reported:

I'm a First Aider. I've been in St John's Ambulance 30 years. She had a blind spot on the eye, paralysis on the opposite side of the damage. It seemed very like either a stroke or thrombosis. She got out of bed to go to the toilet and the other sister found her collapsed on the toilet floor. I sent for assistance to one of the neighbours that's been a nurse. We got her up and I phoned the doctor and he couldn't come so they got an ambulance.

In some cases it was the general practitioner who advised the patient or supporter to call for an ambulance:

I guessed. When we woke up in the morning he said he wanted to go to the toilet – he said 'Pull me up'. I looked at his mouth and it was funny and I thought 'Oh God, he's had a stroke.' I phoned for the doctor and he said get the ambulance straight away. He said it was a stroke.

In several other cases patients and supporters explained that they were unable to reach their general practitioner. In more than 10% of the cases the doctor who came to visit the patient was described as a deputising or 'relief' doctor. The identity of the general practitioner who called was not investigated systematically, but from the statements of patients and supporters it is clear that in less than half of all cases did the patient have any contact with his or her own general practitioner at the time of onset of symptoms. When patients are seen by a deputising doctor this may encourage a cautious response, since nearly all patients with such a contact were referred to hospital. However, referral to hospital is not unusual, and altogether 88% of patients who contacted their general practitioner were admitted to hospital for some time during the first 3 weeks after the stroke.

Thus the proportion of patients admitted to hospital after contacting their general practitioner is higher in this London population than in either Manchester (Brocklehurst *et al.*, 1978*b*) or Bristol (Wade and Langton-Hewer, 1985). In both these studies, as in others (e.g. Askham, 1983; Bamford *et al.*, 1986), there has been a focus of interest on why general practitioners decide to refer a stroke patient for admission to hospital, but little investigation into how and why patients or carers decide to seek medical care in different ways. These results from London indicate that decision-making by patients and supporters is more independent there (i.e. they are more likely to go direct to casualty), probably because hospitals are often more immediately accessible than general practitioners. Both patients and their doctors appear to choose hospitals more often in the urban areas (cf. Bamford *et al.*, 1986), although it seems that there is little benefit for most patients from hospital admission (Wade and Langton-Hewer, 1985). Moreover, this high rate of hospital admission for treatment of stroke is enormously expensive (Wade and Langton-Hewer, 1985). There is a strong argument for developing a community-based service for nursing and rehabilitation. The trial provision of additional home support in the Bristol area was not successful (Wade *et al.*, 1985*a*), but the scheme was small and organised around general practitioners. The reality of coming into care in London suggests that a scheme there should be based around the casualty department, with rapid communication to the patients' general practitioners.

Any scheme for treating more patients at home will depend for its success on the attitudes and inclinations of family doctors (Wade *et al.*, 1985*a*). The general practitioners in Greenwich were asked whether they would like to care for more patients at home, assuming that other community services were available. Only half (52%) of the doctors said they would like to do this; 36% felt they would prefer not to, and 12% made some other comment. Among the observations made by doctors who said they would like to care for more patients at home were caveats about the need for adequate community support:

Oh, I think so. They do better at home than in hospital provided that the services are adequate and the family is there at home.

Perhaps, more surprisingly, there were several doctors who expressed a preference for home care in part because of reservations about hospital care of stroke patients:

I do think that a certain group – the young – should go into hospital, possibly needing surgery. But otherwise much better having people at home – get better more quickly and to be in a geriatric unit is a bit depressing.

No point sending them to hospital so they just rot in there.

They [patients] prefer it. They don't do anything for them in hospital.

They are not getting too much in hospital anyway. In a geriatric ward they start to vegetate.

Other general practitioners indicated that home care was preferable for the doctor as well as for the patient:

For a GP it's a satisfying thing to do. You see the end result. You see the beginning and then when they've got back what they lost.

However, among general practitioners who were generally positive about home care there were also concerns about implications for their workload:

I would be worried about how much time stroke patients would take up. If I had many elderly I would be ambivalent. I know it's preferable from the patient's point of view, and I don't like the way hospital manages them.

The problem of excess workload was also one reason why some doctors were unable to contemplate extending home care for stroke patients:

I couldn't cope with more work.

Not enough time; heavy practice – can't cope with more.

Firstly because circumstances don't allow for it, and furthermore the time. Not enough time.

Other general practitioners considered it was more prudent or practical to refer patients to hospital – for assessment, surgery, nursing care or rehabilitation:

Patients, when they first have a stroke, need really good nursing care; they need to be properly looked after.

Prefer the arrangement at present, especially if there is difficulty walking and anxiety. The idea of getting them in quickly for assessment and then home again works well.

No, I don't think [more home care] is a good idea, I don't think they get the community feeling – the competition with other stroke patients. They are more quickly made independent in hospital.

Altogether, only 10% of the general practitioners reported that they often considered referring a stroke patient aged 65 or over for a specialist neurological assessment. These doctors were also less likely to want to care for more patients at home: only 20% wanted more home care compared with 56% of other doctors who considered specialist neurological assessment less often. Only 3% of the general practitioners said that they often considered the potential for surgery in an older stroke patient, but 75% said they sometimes considered this.

These questions about the attitudes and practices of general practitioners clearly present a diversity of views and opinions. Attitudes to
home or hospital care were not associated with the doctor's training,
country of qualification, number of partners, or workload as indicated by
the number of patients on their list or the proportion of patients in the
practice aged 65 or over. The main characteristic distinguishing doctors
who said they would like to care for more patients at home was age: 61%
of those aged under 50 said they would like to do this compared with 40%
of older doctors. Trainers were less likely to want to give more care at
home (11% compared with 55% of other doctors), and this was not
because they were particularly enthusiastic about hospital services – none
of them reported that they often sought a specialist neurological assessment for older stroke patients.

Regardless of attitudes and preferences, it appears that general practitioners in Greenwich referred patients with stroke to hospital as often, if
not more often, than doctors elsewhere.

Hospital referrals

When patients go to hospital their management may, as Mulley and Arie
(1978) have noted, depend upon bed availability. The wife of a man in his
early sixties had the distressing experience of seeing her desperately ill
husband refused entry at the door of both the main district hospitals:

This came suddenly. His speech started getting a bit slurred and I called the doctor
in. The doctor couldn't get him away yet because the Brook was full and
Greenwich District was full. So he had to wait to see what happened. Then he
went berserk and the doctor came and ordered him away. The only place he could
get him in was the Seaman's. The doctor said he'd had a stroke – a very bad one.

When the general practitioners were asked whether they, in general,
had any difficulty getting a stroke patient admitted to hospital in Greenwich, 17% of them reported that this was often the case, 28% that this
sometimes happened, while 55% said there was never any difficulty.
Single-handed practitioners were more likely to report that they often had
difficulty: 30% of them said this compared with only 11% of doctors in
larger practices. And doctors who qualified in Asia were more likely to
report some problems in getting patients admitted. In part, the problems
of Asian-qualified doctors reflect the high proportion of them who were
single-handed. This difference did persist, though, among doctors in
larger partnerships, but because the numbers are relatively small it was
not statistically significant. (Among doctors in partnerships, 58% of those

who qualified in Asia reported difficulty getting patients admitted, as did 36% of the doctors who qualified elsewhere.)

Among the doctors who had difficulties getting a stroke patient admitted to hospital, 48% of the problems they described were general, 15% were associated with a particular hospital in the health district, and 37% applied to particular patients, almost always specifically to older people with a stroke:

Over 65s, especially if you are asking for an admission under a physician rather than geriatrician.

The older ones. Sometimes you have to have a domiciliary visit to get admission when it is not really necessary.

Geriatric. Very poor service – even for a domiciliary visit one may wait weeks.

The specific difficulties therefore appear to be with the older patients who are the focus of this study. This may be one reason why some of the patients and supporters were advised by their general practitioner to call for an ambulance themselves.

Before considering to which hospital the patients were admitted, it may be illuminating to note what hospital service the general practitioner thought was best for their patients. They were asked whether they had any preferences for a hospital or ward, given that they were seeking to admit a patient aged 70 who had good prospects for survival and rehabilitation. Half of the doctors (53%) said they had a preference and the rest (47%) that they had none; many of the latter group pointed out that they had no choice in the matter since the geriatric services were zoned, with rigid catchment areas for the two main hospitals. Among the doctors expressing a preference, two-thirds of those who specified a ward type would have liked the patient to be admitted to the specialist stroke unit. Doctors appeared to be looking for an interested and energetic service oriented to rehabilitation while not neglecting the medical side. Among the reasons given for preferring the stroke unit were:

Whole-hearted interest in stroke, plus full back-up services. Patients feel things are more likely to be done there than on a geriatric ward.

A positive approach. They really try to get them mobilised and back into the community.

I think they are more likely to have a positive attitude. Stroke patients are seen as an encumbrance on a medical ward and given a low priority.

They get excited about strokes, provide physiotherapy and occupational therapy. Strokes need an aggressive approach.

They know what they are doing. They have the staff. On a general ward [stroke patients] are just stuck in a corner.

Many of the doctors' comments thus reflect the priority they give to a positive approach to the care of stroke patients. Other doctors (about 1 in 6 of those who specified a ward preference) favoured a geriatric ward for a similar reason:

Geriatricians do best – active rehabilitation. Better management of the total person.

Geriatricians are best. Treat them more positively.

A similar number of doctors expressed a preference for care on a medical ward. Again, the main reason appeared to be that, in their experience, treatment on these wards was more positive than elsewhere:

Acute medical rather than geriatric. Treatment is more active. On geriatric wards they are short of staff and geared to not doing much.

Better for morale. If staff not too busy, more is done for them.

With these preferences and observations from the general practitioners in the health district, the experience of the patients may be given some perspective.

In Greenwich, 64% of patients spent all of the first 3 weeks after coming into medical care in hospital, and 30% spent some of that period in hospital. There was little transfer of patients between the hospitals in the acute phase; only 4% of patients had been treated in more than one hospital, and no patients were transferred between the two main district hospitals (except briefly for investigations). Of the patients who went to hospital in the first 3 weeks, 90% received some in-patient care in one or other of the district general hospitals, 10% were admitted to one of the smaller hospitals with geriatric beds, and 4% were treated in a hospital outside the health district.

The way that patients came into care influenced where they were admitted: of the patients who contacted their general practitioner, 57% went to Greenwich District hospital and 24% to the Brook hospital; of those patients who went, or were taken, direct to hospital, 61% went to the Brook and 27% to Greenwich hospital. Thus in one hospital 63% of these admissions were direct through casualty, compared with only 24% at the other main hospital. This difference may reflect bed availability, the status of the Accident and Emergency departments, or, less probably, some characteristics of the different catchment populations. The pattern requires further investigation. The difference in source of admissions appears to explain, in part, why only 40% of the patients at the Brook hospital were aged 75 and over, compared with 70% of patients at Greenwich hospital. No other characteristics of either the patient (sex, marital status, social class) or the stroke (disability, first or subsequent, continence, cognitive impairment or communication loss) were associated with admission to either of the two main hospitals. However, by 3 weeks after the stroke there seemed to have been some selection of seriously disabled patients into the smaller geriatric hospitals: 76% of their patients were rated on the Barthel index as severely or very severely disabled compared with 49% of the patients in the district general hospitals.

In the hospitals there was some movement of patients between wards during the acute phase. Among patients admitted to hospital in the first 3 weeks, 44% had been on a geriatric ward, 54% on a general medical ward, 15% had been admitted (generally transferred from another ward) to the stroke unit, and 7% had been on surgical or other wards. Not surprisingly, those aged 75 or over were more likely than younger patients to be managed on a geriatric ward (59%, compared with 23% of patients aged 60–74). Associated with this age difference, 54% of patients with some urinary incontinence had been on a geriatric ward compared with 37% of patients who were continent. The patient's sex, social class, disability and cognitive impairment were not related to the wards that he or she went to.

Only 25 patients were managed in the stroke unit during the first 3 weeks after the stroke. Possibly because the numbers are small, patients in the stroke unit differed little in most respects from those on other wards. The unit had similar proportions of older and more disabled patients. However, there was some indication that fewer of the stroke unit patients had a problem with comprehension (16% did, compared with 32% of the patients on other wards) or any incontinence of faeces (16% did, compared with 34% elsewhere); these differences were not statistically significant.

Disability 1 month after the stroke

In general, the patients who survived to beyond 3 weeks after the stroke were a relatively disabled group compared, for example, with those in other recent community studies in Bristol (Wade and Langton-Hewer, 1987a) and Oxford (Davies *et al.*, 1989). While few had experienced any severe disability before the stroke, now only a small proportion were independent in all activities of daily living. The comparison of activities

Table 10. *Independence of patients in activities of daily living before the stroke and at the first interview 1 month after the stroke*

Proportion of patients who:	Before the stroke (%)	First interview (%)
Get out of bed without help	95	47
Stand up from chair without help	96	56
Walk 50 yards or more unaccompanied	75	28
Walk up 5 + steps unaccompanied	79	17
Feed themselves without help	94	49
Dress themselves without help	90	38
Groom themselves without help	94	57
Wash body without help	78	21
Cut their toenails themselves	43	11
Use lavatory without help	90	45
No. of patients (= 100%)	162	173

Table 11. *Continence and disability scores of patients at the first interview*

Continence score[b]	Disability score[a]				
	0–4 (%)	5–8 (%)	9–12 (%)	13–16 (%)	All (%)
0	6	0	0	0	2
1	33	4	3	0	14
2	29	21	3	0	15
3	12	25	23	2	14
4	20	50	71	98	55
No. of patients (= 100%)	65	28	35	44	172

[a] The higher the disability score the less severe the disability.
[b] The higher the continence score the less severe the incontinence problem.

before the stroke and at the first interview about 4 weeks after the stroke is shown in Table 10.

Patients with lower (i.e. less able) disability scores (see the Appendix) were much more likely to be incontinent. The relationship between these scores is shown in Table 11, which also documents that at 4 weeks after the stroke 45% of patients had some problem with continence, making this a common and important consequence of stroke (Currie, 1986).

Measures of continence and disability are combined to constitute the

Table 12. *Some characteristics of the patients and their strokes related to Barthel*

Proportion of patients who are/have:	Barthel score					
	0–4 very severe (%)	5–9 severe (%)	10–14 moderate (%)	15–19 mild (%)	20 normal (%)	All patients[a] (%)
Male	39	56	36	35	60	45
Aged 75 or over	74	58	57	52	40	58
Speech problem	83	39	21	22	40	36
Unable to write legibly	89	31	15	9	7	26
Comprehension problem	93	21	11	9	7	27
Orientation score 5 or less	94	33	22	22	7	32
Difficulty with numbers	77	36	43	18	14	33
Hemianopia	68	8	19	9	7	18
Proprioceptive loss	80	30	16	7	0	18
Sensory loss	78	53	33	24	36	42
Abnormal sitting balance	82	38	7	2	0	27
Severe weakness or paralysis of arm	88	42	11	4	0	26
No. of patients (= 100%)	31	52	28	46	15	173

[a] The number for 'all patients' includes one person who was not classified by Barthel score.

Barthel score (Mahoney and Barthel, 1965). As the main measure of disability, the Barthel score was clearly related to clinical measures of impairment and to problems associated with the stroke, as well as to some personal characteristics of the patient. The data are given in Table 12.

This is not an epidemiological study of disability following stroke, since it considers only people aged 60 or over who have survived the acute phase. Nevertheless, the association between features of impairment and functional disability is striking. Although the degree of severity of disability is associated with the proportion of patients with different difficulties it is the multitude of problems facing the group of very severely disabled which is most distinctive. They often have problems of communication, movement, perception and continence together (and, as Chapter 5 will discuss, 58% of these patients died over the following 2 months).

Table 13. *Proportion of patients rated as severely or very severely disabled, by age and sex*

Age	Proportion severely or very severely disabled					
	Men		Women		All	
60–69	44%	(18)[a]	24%	(17)	34%	(35)
70–79	60%	(43)	42%	(43)	51%	(86)
80 +	47%	(15)	56%	(36)	53%	(51)
All patients	54%	(76)	44%	(96)	48%	(172)

[a] Figures in brackets are the numbers on which percentages are based.

Personal characteristics of the patients were not strongly associated with level of disability. There was no association between Barthel score and social class, and although there appears to be some increase with age in the proportion of patients who are severely or very severely disabled this trend is significant only for women patients. The figures are in Table 13, which also shows that among patients aged 60–79 men were more likely to be severely disabled (56%, compared with 37% of women).

Continence was not associated with the patient's sex, but the proportion with any urinary incontinence increased with age, from 23% of patients aged 60–69 to 63% of those aged 80 or over. Age was less markedly associated with incontinence of faeces, but this was a problem among 19% of patients aged 60–74 and 35% of those aged 75 and over. When patients were incontinent a nurse on the ward was asked whether the patient was always aware of this problem; it appeared that a third of the patients were not. Awareness is one of several factors associated with incontinence (Currie, 1986). Not surprisingly, patients with some incontinence had a lower mean score on the assessment of orientation (4.5) compared with continent patients (6.6); and among patients who were unable to complete this assessment (Isaacs and Walkey, 1963) or who gave three or fewer correct responses, 80% had some problem with incontinence.

In general, the measurements of clinical impairment (hemianopia, proprioceptive loss, sensory loss, sitting balance, and arm function: see Appendix) were clearly linked to the severity of disability, but to neither the age nor sex of the patient. However, men were more likely to suffer some proprioceptive loss (26%, compared with 10% of women) and 36% of men had severe or total paralysis of the affected arm compared with

Table 14. *Proportion of patients with weakness at different sites*

	Left side (%)	Right side (%)
Face	17	15
Arm	38	40
Hand	36	39
Leg	46	45

only 18% of women. The proportion of patients with abnormal sitting balance increased with age, from 12% of those aged 60–69 to 36% of patients aged 85 and over.

Disability is generally a result of physical impairment, but, following stroke, patients may have cognitive or perceptual problems which prevent them from initiating and carrying out activities. Altogether 9% of patients had no weakness in their limbs or face when seen at the first interview, but 87% of these patients nevertheless had some disability, usually classified as mild. Thirty-seven per cent of patients had a weakness on their left side, 42% on the right side and 12% on both sides. (The side of the stroke is discussed here in terms of the site of any weakness, not the hemisphere of the lesion in the brain.) The more specific sites of the weakness are shown in Table 14 for 172 patients.

There was no difference in the severity of disability between patients with weakness on the left or right sides, nor was side of the stroke associated with age or sex of the patient, or with the presence of perceptual problems, such as loss of sensation or proprioception. However, patients with right-sided weakness were more disoriented and were, as expected, more likely to have problems with communication. The figures are in Table 15; all differences between left-sided and right-sided strokes are statistically significant, except for 'comprehension'.

Although the problems in communication are assessed crudely in this study, the proportion of patients with speech problems at 4 weeks after stroke is similar to that reported in other studies (Weddell and Beresford, 1979; Wade *et al.*, 1986*a*). Many of these different problems with communication were associated with each other. Problems with expression and comprehension were closely linked: among patients identified as having no speech impairment only 6% were rated as having a problem with comprehension; of those classified as having some problem with expression, 28% were identified as having a problem with understanding; and of the patients with a major speech impairment, 94% also had difficulties

Table 15. *Side of weakness related to communication problems*

	Side of weakness				
	Left (%)	Right (%)	Left + Right (%)	None (%)	All (%)
Expression:					
No problem	79	52	50	86	64
Some problem	14	32	39	14	25
Major problem	7	16	11	0	11
Comprehension:					
No problem	81	72	55	69	73
Some problem	11	17	30	31	18
Major problem	8	11	15	0	9
Writing:					
Legible	86	64	65	79	74
Illegible	7	24	12	14	15
Unable	7	12	23	7	11
Felt had problem with words	21	50	41	43	38
Problem with numbers	16	43	53	29	33
Orientation (Walkey) score 5 or less	19	40	33	43	32
No. of patients (= 100%)	64	72	20	16	172

with comprehension. All the patients who had a major problem expressing themselves said they had a problem with words and failed the 'numbers test' (which was to subtract 7 from 11).

None of the communication problems was associated with the patient's sex, nor were problems with expression or writing associated with the patient's age. However, people aged 75 and over were more likely to have problems with comprehension: 33% did compared with 19% of patients aged 60–74. Difficulties with hearing were, fortunately, not very common, affecting 1 patient in 8; but while all patients aged 60–69 could hear without difficulty, this proportion declined with age, so that fewer than three-fifths of patients aged 85 and over were able to hear without difficulty.

Social class of patients has little relationship to any of the impairments associated with this stage after the stroke. It was not related to orientation, comprehension or expression. However there is one indication that patients from different social classes viewed their problems differently: 26% of middle-class patients and 32% of those classified as working-class were rated as having a problem with expression, but when patients were asked if they had a problem with words (finding or articulating them) only 15% of the patients classified as middle-class thought so, compared with 38% of working-class patients. This finding is difficult to understand; there seems no reason to suppose a greater inclination at this stage to 'denial' among middle-class patients; but 'denial', particularly among speech-impaired patients, is difficult to assess.

Finally, for a relatively high proportion of patients in this study (36%) this was a second or subsequent stroke. These patients with previous experience of stroke were not older than those with first strokes, nor were they more disabled. (Perhaps an older, more disabled group had died in the first 3 weeks.) However, more of the patients with a second or subsequent stroke had communication impairments: 46% of them had difficulties with expression compared with 30% of those with first strokes; and 39% had a problem understanding speech, compared with 20% of patients for whom this was their first stroke.

These impairments and disabilities, particularly in communication and orientation, make it difficult for patients to give valid and reliable responses to questions in an interview. Furthermore some patients in the study (11%) were still too ill at 3 weeks after the stroke for an interview. Altogether about one-quarter of the stroke patients in Greenwich were too ill, disoriented or beset by difficulties in communication to respond adequately to the questionnaire. For these patients information from nurses and supporters has been used to establish events and activities.

Attitudes of patients and supporters to the stroke

As well as suffering the direct effects of the stroke on functioning, many patients shortly after stroke are bewildered and confused about what has happened to them. During the fourth week after the stroke only 63% of the patients in Greenwich (excluding the patients who were too ill or confused to respond) were able to say that they had suffered a stroke. When they were asked 'What is wrong with you? What is your illness called?' 27% said they did not know and 10% said it was something other than stroke. Other conditions mentioned included Parkinson's disease, arthritis, vertigo, heart failure and falls – and usually the patient suffered from this other problem as well. Patients who did not know what was wrong enlarged their response with comments that ranged from 'No idea' and 'Nothing that I can think of', to 'I can't say – seems as if I just faded away' and descriptions of symptoms to which they were unable to give a name:

Loss of power on the left side – I don't know the medical name.

Well as far as I know it's my balance and my movement. I don't know what they call it – they just say you are doing very well.

Many of the patients who did not know their diagnosis appeared relatively unconcerned; others felt it was time they knew:

Wish they'd tell me. They take blood tests and X-rays, but they don't tell me what's up.

That's what I'd like to know. I must have gone funny in the head.

Knowing the diagnosis was clearly less likely if the patient was disoriented: only 29% of patients with a Walkey score (orientation score: see Appendix) of less than 6 reported that their illness was a stroke, compared with 73% of those with a Walkey score of 6–8. Older patients were less likely to say they had had a stroke; the proportion saying this fell from 80% of patients aged 60–69, to 51% of those aged 80 or over, and this trend persisted even among patients who were well oriented (score of 7 or 8 on the Walkey scale). The proportion who knew they had suffered a stroke was not associated with the sex or social class of the patient, nor with previous experience of a stroke or reporting a chronic illness; but patients whose disability after the stroke was mild or non existent were more likely to know (74% did, compared with 55% of patients with more severe disability).

Only 7 supporters (5%) failed to report that the patient's illness was a stroke. Of these, 3 described the illness as an accident or a fall, the others as Parkinson's disease, pneumonia, a strangulated hernia, and salmonella poisoning (although in this last case the patient reported the illness as a stroke).

Patients and supporters were asked for their evaluation of the illness as 'serious, mild or something in between'. The responses, presented in Table 16, show that supporters took a more serious view of the illness; and while 94% of supporters said they were concerned 'a lot' by the illness, only 61% of the patients said this and 26% described themselves as concerned only 'a little' or 'not at all'.

Rating of disability and the supporter's perception of the severity of the illness were closely related; the proportion describing the illness as serious

Table 16. *Views of patients and supporters on the severity of the illness*

Illness described as:	Supporters (%)	Patients (%)
Serious	71	41
In between	20	30
Mild	9	29
No. of people (= 100%)	142	119

declined from 85% when the patient's disability was classified as very severe to 46% when the patient was classified as normal. However, only 45% of the patients whose disability was classified as severe or very severe regarded the illness as serious. These patients tended to reflect on the stroke in relative terms: in comparison with previous experience ('When I think about the stroke my husband had'; 'Not so serious as the last one'), with the situation of others ('Mild compared with what I've seen on the ward'), or in relation to recovery already made (an 'in between' illness 'because when I first came in here I was pretty ill then, but I've recovered from that. I looked pale and drawn but I've got colour now'; 'because ... my hands came back, my legs came back'). Older patients tended to view the illness as less serious; 42% of patients aged 75 or over described the illness as mild compared with 18% of younger patients.

Expectations for recovery

Taken altogether, patients appeared to have a more optimistic view of the stroke than the supporters. Their views on recovery in the first 3 or 4 weeks and their expectations for future recovery are shown in Table 17.

Patients' expectations for recovery were not related to sex, age or social class, but patients who were more disabled expected less recovery; the proportion expecting 'a lot' of recovery declined from 69% of patients classified as independent to 42% of patients with severe or very severe disability. Only 16% of the supporters of patients with moderate or more severe disability expected the patient to make 'a lot' of recovery; 15% did not expect any further improvement.

Most patients felt that, 4 weeks after the stroke, they could contribute significantly to their own recovery; 39% felt they could do a lot to help themselves, 34% that they could give some help, 13% a little, 5% nothing, while 9% said they did not know. Essentially patients described three

Table 17. *Attitudes of patients and supporters to the patient's recovery*

	Recovery so far		Expect to recover	
Degree of recovery	Patients (%)	Supporters (%)	Patients (%)	Supporters (%)
A lot	48	40	52	20
Some	28	19	17	31
A little	16	27	6	17
Not at all	7	12	9	14
Don't know	1	2	16	18
No. of people (= 100%)	123	144	117	144

general ways in which they could help themselves: by following the advice of doctors and therapists; by building upon their own willpower and determination; and by changing their circumstances, for example by leaving the protectiveness of hospital or having adaptations made at home. Some patients were concerned that their own potential for recovery was not being constructively developed. Two severely disabled men in their seventies and in hospital illustrate this problem:

Well, they'll always tell you here you know, you must help yourself – but you couldn't always understand what that entails. I don't really know how I can help myself. Not being more of a nuisance than you can to help the nurses and so on?

Once they tell us what to do a ruddy lot. But at the moment you don't know what's best to get you better.

However, the general spirit was that the patients felt they could help themselves and they were getting on with it:

You try to do what you can yourself, as you should, and doctors give help. Can't wait all the time for the doctors. Got to help yourself.

These attitudes to helping themselves were not related to the patient's age, sex, social class or perception of the illness severity; but more disabled patients were less likely to feel they could help their recovery a lot, the proportion saying this falling from 50% of the patients classified (on Barthel scores) as normal to only 25% among patients who were categorised as being very severely disabled. The patient's emotional distress appears to exert a consistent effect in the sense that patients who were more distressed were less likely to feel they could do a lot to help their recovery: the proportion saying this fell from 62% of patients who made no positive responses on the 'emotional distress' dimension of the Nottingham Health Profile (see Appendix) to only 19% of those who agreed with six or more of the statements. Insofar as the Profile is an indicator of depressed mood (Ebrahim *et al.*, 1986) this is not surprising. It was noticeable, however, that while many patients mentioned the positive side of their mental resources (e.g. determination, willpower) very few alluded to any barriers caused by emotional distress. (And probably some of those who were most distressed did not answer the question.)

The supporters in particular, when considering how the patient could help himself or herself, emphasised willpower and positive attitudes. However, they were somewhat more cautious than the patients, and when they said that the patient could help 'a lot' or 'some' (see Table 18 for proportions) they often added caveats. The daughter of a 70-year-old woman with mild disability but relatively high emotional distress, commented:

If she wasn't so depressed. She feels useless that she can't do anything anymore. If she had a more definite aim in life she could do a lot to help herself if she would; instead of thinking she's on her way out.

And the daughter of a recently bereaved man who was living in his own home, pointed to the important question: why bother helping yourself?

If he puts his mind to it. He's lacking mental and physical activity at the moment. He hasn't got the incentive now [patient's wife] is not there.

Supporters' attitudes to patients helping themselves were clearly related to measures of the patient's mental state: the proportion of supporters who thought the patient could do a lot to help recovery was 50% for patients with 5 or more correct responses on the test of cognition and orientation (see Appendix) but only 26% for those with a lower score; and this proportion was 56% among patients scoring 0 to 5 on the 'emotional distress' element of the Nottingham Health Profile, falling to only 21% for supporters of patients with a higher score.

Supporters' views were not as clearly associated with the patient's physical disability as had been the case for patients' views. The main distinction in supporters' views was between how much they felt patients with very severe disability could do, and the rest; only 15% of the former group were described as being able to do a lot to help their recovery compared with 45% of other patients.

Both patients and supporters seemed to feel that patients aged 80 and over were less able to do a lot to help their recovery, but this difference was not statistically significant. However, 12% of the supporters of patients aged 60–79 felt that the patient could do nothing to help his or her

Table 18. *Supporters' views on the extent to which different people can help the patient's recovery*

Can help recovery:	Doctors, nurses, therapists (%)	Patient (%)	Supporter (%)
A lot	30	41	21
Some	20	25	47
Just a little	20	12	14
Not at all	15	19	14
Don't know	15	3	4
No. of supporters (= 100%)	144	144	144

recovery compared with 35% of the supporters of patients aged 80 or over. Other characteristics of the patient – sex, social class – did not differentiate the views of supporters.

The views of supporters, at 4 weeks after stroke, about how much they, the patients, and medical or rehabilitation therapists could contribute to the patients' recovery are shown in Table 18.

As with their views on what patients could do, the supporters were likely to feel they could do less to help patients aged 80 or over to recover; 44% thought they could do little or nothing to help if the patient was in this oldest age group, compared with 21% of the supporters of patients aged 60–79. The supporters' views were not associated with whether or not they and the patient normally lived together, or with their family relationship to each other. However, the supporters' rating of the quality of their relationship with the patient before the stroke was a factor; 76% of supporters who described this relationship as 'very happy' thought they could do 'a lot' or 'some' to help, compared with only 54% of supporters who felt the relationship had been only 'fairly happy' or 'not happy'. This finding becomes more comprehensible when one considers what it was that supporters felt they could do to help. Carers offered several different kinds of support – emotional, social and, to a lesser extent, practical – but it was mainly psychosocial support and 'caring understanding'.

Several supporters, in the following cases all daughters or sons of the patient, referred to that special resource in some close relationships:

Family love – he's being looked after, he's being protected; he's not abandoned like those at the hospital.

One daughter described her love as if prescribed by the doctors. She felt she could help 'some':

Just by giving her the love that they've told me to give her.

But the daughter of another patient felt there was nothing she could do:

Apart from giving her lots of love and going to see her I can't do anything positive.

It may be relevant that in these cases of offering 'love' the patients were mentally confused. With other disabled patients the hope and encouragement was sometimes more active. The son of one woman who seemed only slightly disoriented felt he could do 'just a little' to help recovery by:

Visiting her – goading her and really pushing her because she would just lay back and do nothing.

Much of this support was designed to respond to problems seen in the patient such as depression, hopelessness and lack of confidence. Other problems that the supporters felt patients had (especially male patients it appeared) were related to social isolation, lack of companionship and lack of meaningful social involvement. These were viewed, in this context, as barriers to the patient's recovery and supporters sought to bridge the gaps by making the patients feel wanted, important and part of everyday life outside the 'sick room'. Two women illustrated how they thought they could give 'some' help to their husbands' recovery:

I do daily visits thinking this helps him to feel wanted; I still talk to him about affairs and what needs to be paid. It helps him to think he is still master of his house, that sort of thing.

By greater encouragement and acting positively in his company and involving him in decision making.

Several supporters felt that their visits were important, both to let patients know that someone cared for their company and to give meaning to days which were often quite empty. The wife of a man who had been very active in voluntary organisations before the stroke emphasised this point:

I help him all I can, cheer him up, feed him up! If you keep a sense of companionship – that's the most important; an attitude of caring.

In general, supporters said they would do all they possibly could for the patient, but few referred to any specific practical or therapeutic tasks. There was scant reference to helping in the patient's formal rehabilitation (referred to only by the carers of two patients with aphasia), but a small number of carers had their own approaches to helping recovery:

By going and seeing him and giving him the encouragement he needs. I'm doing everything possible. I'll get him a tennis ball to help him get the use of his fingers.

And a daughter-in-law of a woman at home sought to link her efforts at rehabilitation to the patient's interests before the stroke:

I got her a tapestry to do and tried her with a jig-saw which she found difficult ... Trying to stimulate her mind and get her interested in things; and trying different things to help her hand – to improve the grip, that sort of thing.

The supporters had relatively modest expectations about the extent to which doctors and rehabilitation therapists could affect recovery.

They are lovely people, but they can't work miracles. He couldn't wish for better care – but what can they do?

There's not much they can do. Medical abilities don't really come into it. There's no cure.

In considering help from doctors and therapists, several supporters emphasised the psychological consequences of the stroke and the need for emotional support. The daughter of a woman who was very distressed by a stroke which caused mild disability felt:

One of the things I think the medical staff have not been very good at has been on the psychological side. They haven't really kept me or her enough informed. Because she is intelligent [was head of English teaching], because her intelligence and speech are not impaired she would do better if they explained more to her what was happening. It would help with this appalling depression and it would certainly help me, if for example, they were to make an occasion when we could all sit down and discuss it together.

Similar observations were made by the supporters of patients at home, as well as those in hospital.

They could make her existence a little happier. It would help her psychologically to see a doctor every so often. The doctors don't worry about her. Her old doctor used to come in once a fortnight but these other two don't bother.

Parallel with their higher expectations for recovery, patients appeared more generally optimistic about the contribution that rehabilitation could make to their recovery. In a subsample of 50 patients who were asked directly, 60% said they thought the doctors, therapists and nurses could do a lot to help their recovery, and several were impatient for more help:

Well I think they're helping you all the time. I'd be ruddy glad if they'd send me to this ward where you had to do the stroke exercises all the time – give you something to do.

That's one of the things I want to find out. I want to get into the stroke unit. The whole object of the exercise is for me to get cured in double-quick time. There's a good chance you'll come and see me again in two months time and nothing will have happened – no services received. I want a unit where I can go and do therapy.

The next chapter looks at the patients who did and did not receive rehabilitation, considers the attitudes of patients and their supporters to the care received, and makes some assessment of the contribution of therapy to recovery.

SUMMARY

Coming into care The experience of stroke among these survivors did not follow the typical scenario of sudden loss of function and immediate efforts to consult with the general practitioner. Five-sixths of patients were at home when they first noticed symptoms of the stroke, which most then sought to understand through consultation with family and friends. About one-fifth of these patients were too ill to play any role in seeking medical help. Altogether, among patients in the community, 40% ultimately went, or were taken, direct to hospital. This high proportion was clearly related to the patient's social class, increasing from none of the patients in social classes 1 and 2 to 59% of patients in social class 5. Characteristics of the stroke, other than loss of speech, were not related to seeking help from the general practitioner. The time and place when symptoms began, as well as expectations about the help from their general practitioner, appeared to influence the response of patients and their families. The way that patients came into hospital care, direct or through their general practitioner, influenced the choice of hospital in which they were treated. In Greenwich, 64% of patients spent all of the first 3 weeks in hospital. Patients in geriatric, general medical or stroke unit beds were differentiated mainly by age and continence. This process of coming into care has important implications for the costs, if not the effectiveness, of care. Half the general practitioners in the health district indicated that they would prefer to care for more patients at home.

Disability These survivors were a relatively disabled group: for example, the proportion who dressed without help fell from 90% before the stroke to 38% at 1 month after the stroke. At the first interview nearly half the patients had some incontinence, which was especially common among more disabled and older patients. Among patients aged 60–79,

56% of men compared with 37% of women were classified by their Barthel scores as severely disabled. Patients rated as having very severe disability had a distinctive clustering of the problems of communication, movement, perception and continence. Nearly a quarter of all the patients were too communication-impaired, ill or disoriented for an interview. However, even among patients able to respond, only 63% reported that they had suffered a stroke. Nearly all the supporters were aware of the diagnosis and, on the whole, they viewed the illness as more severe than did the patients.

Recovery   Supporters had a more pessimistic view about recovery and prospects in rehabilitation. Both patients with more severe disability and their supporters expected less recovery than others. The supporters had generally modest expectations about the contribution that health care could make to recovery; they were also more cautious about the extent to which they felt patients could help themselves to recover.

A number of supporters alluded to psychological problems as barriers to the patient's recovery, and supporters frequently discussed their own help in terms of giving emotional or social support and 'caring understanding'. Few supporters referred to helping with specific therapeutic tasks or to being involved in the patient's formal rehabilitation.

CHAPTER FOUR

Hospital care and rehabilitation

Most stroke patients spend some time in hospital, but almost nothing is known about their daily experiences there, about their attitudes to care and to hospital life, or about their main worries, concerns or aspirations. This curious vacuum in information may reflect considerable hesitation among professionals about how much they want to know, and an ambivalence and uncertainty among doctors, therapists and nurses about what they can do that will improve the lives of stroke patients. Medical attitudes to the management of stroke and to rehabilitation appear to have been characterised by an 'air of pessimism'. It has been suggested that stroke inspires 'therapeutic nihilism' (Norris and Hachinski, 1982) and that, in general, doctors exhibit a lack of interest in stroke rehabilitation: '[it] is often considered to be something that other people do when the doctor has become therapeutically bankrupt ... the suggestion has been made that patients should not be subject to unwanted activity but be left in peace to die in dignity' (Mulley, 1981, p. 24). In a study of the management at home of stroke patients, Isaacs and colleagues (1976) found that general practitioners made a limited contribution; this they attributed, in part, to the pessimistic attitude to stroke rehabilitation which prevailed in hospitals at the time when these doctors received their training. There are no data about the current attitudes of either general practitioners or hospital doctors, although the development of stroke units suggests that some doctors at least may have more optimistic views. This chapter looks in detail at the rehabilitation received by patients and at its effects. It begins, though, with the patients' views on life in hospital.

What patients liked and disliked about hospital life

At the second interview 9 months after the stroke patients were asked whether there was anything about their experience in hospital which especially pleased them, and if there was anything which especially upset them.

About two-thirds of patients reported something about their hospital experience which especially pleased them, most commonly (about a third of all patients) that the staff, particularly nurses, had been so kind, caring and encouraging. A woman who had spent 3 weeks in a geriatric ward said:

They were very kind, very gentle, always bright and cheerful – first thing in the morning. I used to admire them all for that, the domestic staff as well as the nurses.

As in studies of general practitioners (Cartwright, 1964), the personal qualities, concern and communication, rather than technical effectiveness, are the characteristics mentioned most commonly about hospital staff. Communication may be taken to embrace everything from sitting and chatting to patiently explaining matters. A man with severe disability described his single pleasure in hospital as:

Only the goodness of the heart of the staff; they were very nice sitting and talking to you.

No patient explicitly mentioned the explanation and advice given by staff, but about 1 in 8 made some specific reference to the encouragement and effort of the therapists. A man who was on the stroke unit for more than 4 months said:

I enjoyed myself in there; they were so nice to you, those physiotherapists and that. One of them was like a mother to me; nothing they wouldn't do for you. They gave me bits and pieces to make everything easier. They always used to talk with you. Sister came in every morning to talk with me.

Several patients commented on the unstinting work of the staff – sometimes surprised by how much had to be done:

The way they worked and the tireless way they did things for you. I realised how much they had to do, but their lot was very hard.

There were very few positive comments about organisational or structural characteristics of the hospital. However, five patients commented positively about the food in hospital. One man who lived alone in a chaotic council flat reported that nothing pleased him especially, but:

I was contented in hospital. I had people to speak to and I had my meals. It seemed a bit of comfort.

But 2 of the patients appeared to praise the food in lieu of anything else positive to say:

The grub was lovely. Nothing [else] pleased me in hospital.

This hospital, you get good food. I've never been in hospital [before]. I couldn't say I liked it.

Altogether, one-third of patients were unable to think of anything which pleased them; several indicated that, for them, being a dependent patient in hospital had no positive aspects. It could mean loss of control over daily habits and the company of strangers. A man of 78 who spent 5 weeks in hospital said:

Well, I was glad to get out of the hospital. They put me in a geriatric ward and there was six in there. They couldn't help it, but you couldn't hold a conversation with any of them.

And another man aged 67 who spent 2 months in the other district hospital said he could not think of any encouraging aspects:

When I was on [medical ward] it was alright; you used to get more attention. Down the other place [on the geriatric ward] it was like a prison. I sat 15 hours a day looking at a wall. We used to have argument after argument. I never used to get no training on that ward.

These themes of social isolation on the ward and lack of therapy were each taken up by 5% of patients as particular aspects of hospital life that had upset them. A former boxing champion, aged 75, commented:

When I was in the geriatric ward I felt too young to be in there. I was fed up in there. Everywhere you looked there was no one to talk to. All I could do was read. I mean there's old and old.

And a woman in her mid-sixties who had spent 2 weeks on a general medical ward said:

These little small wards with only six beds – no company. I don't like the atmosphere of the place ... I couldn't get out of there, it was depressing.

Altogether, fewer than half of the patients identified something about their experience in hospital which especially upset them. One problem, however, was mentioned by 1 in 7 of all the patients and was easily the most common complaint: getting help from the nurses, particularly for the toilet and particularly at night:

We had an episode about [diarrhoea], because they didn't seem to be doing much about it until my husband got shirty. In the end with not being able to get out of bed, it got bad; I was in tears. It was getting me down. Nights were the worst because you know the old night-sisters they couldn't care less. You'd want to call them, ring for them, but it was terrible.

And a woman patient in the other main hospital said:

Don't like those places. Night time when you wanted the commode, you'd ask for it and it would be such a long time to get it.

For the dependent patient who needs help to use the toilet at night the various tensions, including not wishing to wake everyone else, seem to leave a depressing memory. Of course, during the day its different – at least you can make a noise:

All the urinals were down the women's end. You could shout all day and never get any attention. I don't like to criticise the nurses because they are very busy, but I shouted all day and no one would come to see you. It was terrible. When I left there was no doctor or sister to say cheerio. They were glad to see the back of me and I was glad to get out.

It was clearly difficult for some patients to negotiate a new *modus vivendi* in the hospital, and relations with the staff providing most of the everyday support seem to have been precarious. A 67-year old woman who needed help to wash and dress reported:

I was very happy when I went to hospital ... it was the shock of having to ask people to do things for you. And they seemed to think you were malingering, that you could do more for yourself. The nurses seemed to think you were a bit of a nuisance. One nurse came and told me to say 'thank you'.

Unfortunately, the unhappy experience with a single nurse soured the memories of the oldest patient in the study:

There was only one thing: at night one of the nurses, I don't know if she didn't like me, but she did curse me. I dreaded the nights when she was on. If I couldn't lift myself she says 'You can, you're not ill'. And I wonder what am I here for.

The problem of striking a balance between being too protective and pressing the patients too hard applies in hospital as well as at home. Both patients and nurses may find policies for maintaining independence quite trying:

Well, there was always an argument when I wanted my colostomy bag changed. I suppose they wanted to keep me active as regards that. They'd insist on getting me to try to do it myself.

Nurses appear to be the key figures influencing the quality of the patient's stay in hospital. It is likely that more comforting, counselling and communication are provided to stroke patients by nursing staff than by any other group in the hospital; they spend more time with patients than any other group, and may be most knowledgeable about problems associated with bowels and bladder, emotions (especially early in the morning and late at night) and diet. 'Yet very little has been written about the nurse's role in rehabilitation and there have been strikingly few surveys of nursing skills and their relationship to the quality of the patient's life' (Mulley, 1981, p. 32). Christie and Lawrence (1978), interviewing stroke patients discharged from an Australian hospital, report that generally positive attitudes were expressed towards nurses, although nurses were viewed as less important than doctors, from whom patients expected information about themselves, their illness and their future. Altogether, nurses appear to be the most critical element in the patient's experience of daily life in hospital. The balance between their expressions of interest and indifference may have a profound effect on patients' attitudes to the stroke and to themselves.

Rehabilitation in hospital

On the whole, as was indicated in the previous chapter, patients and their families are looking to rehabilitation as the main treatment that will restore independence after stroke. Many professionals, on the other hand, exhibit a lack of enthusiasm for rehabilitation due to a lack of evidence that rehabilitation works. It may be doing no harm, but is it doing any good? For many years rehabilitation has been tried with stroke patients without systematic research to evaluate the outcome. This situation is changing, although the design of adequate studies to assess the success of rehabilitation is fraught with difficulties (Hewer, 1976; Forer and Miller, 1980), not least that of establishing agreement on appropriate indicators of outcome.

Granger and colleagues (1979) have described the objectives of rehabilitation in terms of maintaining medical stability, improving functional status, and assisting the family and patient in adjusting to any residual long-term disability. Other specialists in rehabilitation have emphasised the difference between the aims of acute care and those of rehabilitation. 'It is not the length of time that a stroke patient survives that determines whether rehabilitation is significant. Rather it is the quality of life during that period of survival. Factors which contribute to the quality of life for the stroke patient and can be enhanced by rehabilitation are: independence in self-care, living at home or outside an institution and involvement in employment, homemaking or some type of daily activity' (Anderson *et al.*, 1979, p. 107). However, when outcomes have been measured they have typically been limited to one aspect such as self-care (ADL: activities of daily living) or return to work; and it has proved difficult, given differences in settings, rehabilitation regimes and measurements of outcome, to make statements about the general benefits of rehabilitation.

The contribution of rehabilitation is considered for patients in Greenwich by looking at who received therapy, what patients thought of this, and what difference it made to the performance of activities of daily living. The experience of speech therapy is considered in a separate section below.

Who receives therapy?

Great care was needed to establish which patients received which type of support in the first weeks after the stroke. Patients sometimes could not distinguish speech therapy from occupational therapy, and there were instances when, for example, making tea or participating in group activities were not understood as occupational therapy. It was especially difficult to use reports from speech-impaired patients about receipt of speech therapy – their responses sometimes contradicted one's own observations. The therapies were often individually tailored and varied in frequency depending upon the patient's condition. Use of therapy is quantified here solely in terms of whether the patient received any active therapy beyond an initial assessment. The classification is based upon observation, reports from patients and from nurses and checking of the ward records.

Altogether 81% of patients had received physiotherapy in the period before the first interview, and 42% had received occupational therapy. This pattern, in which about twice as many patients have physical as compared with occupational therapy during the acute phase of the stroke, has been found in other parts of the country (e.g. Oxfordshire: Davies *et al.*, 1989; on the medical units in the Edinburgh stroke trial: Garraway *et al.*, 1980*b*), although the difference was greater in South Manchester (Brocklehurst *et al.*, 1978*c*). The proportion of patients who have remedial therapy is obviously limited by the availability of services, particularly in the community, and this is illustrated by differences between patients who are managed at home and those in hospital. In Greenwich there was only one domiciliary therapist treating patients with any conditions, so few of the patients at home received formal therapy (the figures are in Table 19). The proportion receiving therapy at home differed little from the situation in Oxfordshire, where almost half the patients were being managed at home by the general practitioner (Davies *et al.*, 1989).

Among patients in hospital there was no significant difference in the likelihood of receiving physiotherapy or occupational therapy between patients admitted to the different hospitals or between those on general

Table 19. *Patients' place of care and receipt of remedial therapy during the first 3 weeks after the stroke*

Patient received:	Patient at:			
	Home	Home and hospital	Hospital	All
Physiotherapy	18% (11)[a]	69% (49)	93% (108)	81% (168)
Occupational therapy	9% (11)	38% (48)	47% (109)	42% (168)

[a] Figures in brackets are the numbers on which the percentages are based.

medicine and geriatric wards. However, as in the Edinburgh stroke trial (Garraway *et al.*, 1980*b*), patients admitted to the stroke unit were more likely to have occupational therapy in the acute phase: 80% of them did compared with 36% of patients on other wards. In one sense at least the perception of several patients that more rehabilitation was going on elsewhere was correct.

Access to rehabilitation was not related to the patient's age or sex, nor to the side of the stroke or whether this was a first stroke. However, the patients who had physiotherapy and those who had occupational therapy differed from each other in several respects, the principal one apparently being that those having occupational therapy were a less disabled group. The distribution of the therapies between patients with different levels of severity of disability is similar to that found in the European study (Aho *et al.*, 1980) with some focus upon middle-range disability rather than the concentration of therapy on those in the worst state which was reported in the Manchester (Brocklehurst *et al.*, 1978*c*) and Oxfordshire (Davies *et al.*, 1989) studies. However, the provision of physiotherapy appears to be targeted on those patients with greater disability and on those whose impairments include visuospatial and sensory disorders. The figures are shown in Table 20. The relatively early focus of physiotherapy on patients with severe disabilities is probably intended to prevent secondary complications and spasticity. This provides the platform for subsequently improving function and for involvement of occupational therapists.

Clearly occupational therapy was less likely to be given to patients who were incontinent and to those at the extremes of disability, either mild or severe. There is no evidence that occupational therapy was directed in particular at patients with perceptual or sensory deficits (and those with left hemianopia received less); it probably makes sense that until patients reach a certain level of competence (for example, achieving sitting balance), physiotherapy should be the dominant form of rehabilitation to

Table 20. *Patients' use of rehabilitation related to severity of disability and specific impairments*

	Proportion who received:		No. of patients (= 100%)
	Physiotherapy (%)	Occupational therapy (%)	
Barthel (disability) grade:			
Very severe	83	10	31
Severe	88	49	52
Moderate	89	57	28
Mild	77	56	44
Normal	50	14	14
Incontinence:			
Urine			
Yes	87	26	72
No	77	54	96
Faeces			
Yes	88	22	49
No	79	50	119
Clinical features:			
Hemianopia			
None	79	46	126
Left	100	13	15
Right	100	58	12
Proprioception			
Normal	75	49	106
Loss	95	50	22
Sitting balance			
Normal	78	50	118
Abnormal	89	20	45
Hand sensation			
Normal	76	43	87
Reduced	83	51	47
None	100	38	16
Arm function			
Normal	68	43	40
Slight/moderate weakness	80	49	
Severe weakness	92	41	39

be followed by occupational therapy. However, in Greenwich few patients (10) began occupational therapy after the first interview, and only 4 patients began physiotherapy later than the first weeks. Although it is argued that almost no recovery occurs after 6 months (Brocklehurst *et al.*, 1978a), at the time of the second interview 13% of patients were

Table 21. *Receipt of rehabilitation by patients who are 'good prospects'*

Patient unable to manage:	Proportion who received:	
	Occupational therapy	Physiotherapy
Bed transfer	53% (60)[a]	89% (61)
Chair transfer	53% (49)	92% (50)
Walking 50 yards independently	54% (87)	85% (87)
Stairs	56% (103)	88% (105)
Feeding self	49% (57)	93% (58)
Dressing	48% (75)	89% (75)
Grooming	46% (41)	88% (41)
Bathing	49% (104)	88% (104)
Toilet	49% (57)	90% (58)

[a] Numbers in brackets are the number of dependent patients.

having physiotherapy, all but one of whom had begun treatment in the first few weeks; and 16% of patients were attending for occupational therapy, two-thirds of whom had begun therapy before the first interview. So in Greenwich, as elsewhere (Brocklehurst *et al.*, 1978*c*; Garraway *et al.*, 1980*b*), the pattern of use of remedial therapy is established early after the stroke. It appears that physiotherapy focuses on those with most impairment, while occupational therapy is given more to the patients with good prospects for recovery.

Over the first 6 months after the stroke a third of the patients who had physiotherapy died, as did one-fifth of the patients who had received occupational therapy in the first few weeks. Patients with more severe disability were much more likely to die before 6 months, the proportion increasing from 9% of those with mild or no disability 1 month after the stroke to 68% of the patients with very severe disability. Patients with low Barthel scores at 1 month after the stroke appear to have a poor prognosis for survival and recovery of function (Wade and Langton Hewer, 1987*a*). Patients who are dependent in some way but who have Barthel scores of 5 or more may be considered 'good prospects' for survival; perhaps they should be a focus for early rehabilitation. Among those in this group who were dependent in different respects, the proportions receiving remedial therapy in the acute phase are shown in Table 21.

In general, among the 'good prospects', there was little difference in the ability to do things independently between those who received remedial therapy and those who did not. The only differences were that 78% of those who received occupational therapy needed help to bathe compared with 93% of those who did not (a finding opposite to that expected), while

88% of those having physiotherapy were unable to bathe compared with 68% of patients not receiving physiotherapy. The corresponding figures for eating independently were 52% and 21%. There was therefore little specificity about the use of remedial therapy for patients with different functional limitations; and, for example, even among 'good prospects' only half of those who were dependent in self-care were receiving occupational therapy.

The effects of rehabilitation

Does the situation described above matter? It would if those who received therapy benefited from it. It would then seem appropriate to argue, as others have done (Brocklehurst *et al.*, 1978c; Davies *et al.*, 1989), for reconsidering the criteria of selection of patients for remedial therapy, so that priority was given more to patients with good prospects for recovery and less to those who were likely to die. However, for many years the research on the effectiveness of therapy has produced equivocal and ultimately inconclusive results, not least because of a lack of agreement on appropriate indicators of outcome and, following this, a lack of sensitive methodological tools for assessing outcome.

The comparison of results from different studies of rehabilitation is generally not valid because of differences in settings, rehabilitation regimes and measurement of outcome. Taken at face value such comparisons are not very illuminating: studies of functional ability among patients with and without rehabilitation have indicated both little or no benefit (Feldman *et al.*, 1962; Peacock *et al.*, 1972) and substantial advantage (Lehmann *et al.*, 1975) among patients receiving rehabilitation. More recent reports from American rehabilitation centres have been more consistently positive about the value of stroke rehabilitation (Feigenson *et al.*, 1979); Anderson and colleagues (1979) report that 'Rehabilitation did not significantly lengthen the duration of survival from onset to interview or death but rather had its principal effect on the quality of life during survival' (p. 107). However, these recent studies are based upon outcomes for selected stroke survivors referred to rehabilitation centres, and do not generally involve any randomisation of patients.

One randomised controlled trial of (out-patient) physiotherapy has been reported (D. S. Smith *et al.*, 1981). Between 1972 and 1978, 121 patients with a recently confirmed stroke who had been admitted to Northwick Park Hospital in Middlesex (only 11% of all stroke admissions were considered suitable) were randomly allocated to one of three treatment regimens: intensive therapy given 4 whole days a week, conventional therapy involving attendance 3 half-days a week or no routine rehabilitation. Outcome was assessed on the basis of ability to carry out activities of daily living, and was measured at discharge and at 3, 6 and 12 months after entry into the trial. In short, the results indicated that decreasing amounts of treatment were associated with a greater tendency to deteriorate. Some patients in all three groups improved in the activities of daily living, and when patients who deteriorated are excluded from analyses, the differences in degree of improvement are not significant between the three groups. In conclusion, the authors suggest that a small proportion of stroke patients are suitable for intensive out-patient rehabilitation, and that this would be effective for these patients. However, 'We cannot be sure which parts of the overall regimen – physiotherapy, occupational therapy or non-specific care and attention – were responsible for the observed improvement apparently associated with active treatment. This is a subject for further trials' (D. S. Smith *et al.*, 1981, p. 519).

The average interval between stroke and entry to the trial was 5–6 weeks. This is probably later than the optimal time to begin therapy to capitalise upon spontaneous recovery (Andrews, 1978); and the amount of in-patient therapy received by patients is not specified. The average level of disability among patients admitted to the trial was not high; as the authors note, the possibility that this was due to intensive in-patient rehabilitation indicates the need for trials starting immediately after the stroke.

The relationship between intensity of therapy and functional outcome was not confirmed in a study of a less selected group of patients; Wade and colleagues (1984) concluded that studies should consider the timing and content of therapy, as well as its intensity.

In Edinburgh, Garraway and colleagues (1980*a, b*) have compared functional outcome between patients randomly allocated to a stroke unit and to medical units. Patients in the stroke unit were more likely to receive physiotherapy and occupational therapy, and to have a significantly shorter delay between admission to hospital and the start of these therapies. When outcome was assessed at a mean of 60 days after admission to hospital, 62% of survivors from the stroke unit were rated as independent compared with 45% of the survivors from medical units; therefore 'the stroke unit improved the natural history of stroke by increasing the proportion of patients who were returned to functional independence' (Garraway *et al.*, 1980*b*, p. 1040). However, 1 year after the initial assessment the difference between survivors from the stroke unit and the medical units had disappeared. Garraway and colleagues (1980*a*) suggest that the disappearance of the advantage held by patients from the stroke unit may have been due to overprotection by the families of patients who had been treated in the stroke unit and to early discharge from medical units of patients whose full rehabilitation potential had been realised.

On the basis of assessment shortly after discharge from hospital it appeared that independent patients from the stroke unit were receiving more family assistance than independent patients from medical units; and dependent patients from medical units were allowed to do more than similar patients from the stroke unit (Garraway, *et al.*, 1980*a*). There is supporting evidence from elsewhere that stroke patients frequently do less than they are able to (Sheikh *et al.*, 1979) and that the chief carer may be unaware of the patient's ability to perform some activities (Andrews, 1978). It is surprising, however, that the 'problem' of overprotectiveness should be greater among patients from the stroke unit, when the relatives and friends of patients from the stroke unit both had more contact with hospital staff and were more satisfied with communication with these staff than were the relatives of patients from the medical units (Murray *et al.*, 1982). Thus the families of patients on the stroke unit had more opportunity to be involved in hospital rehabilitation and preparation for the future; 'the reasons why families might have adopted a more protective role to the detriment of the long-term functional outcome of these patients are not known' (Garraway *et al.*, 1980*a*).

Possibly the alternative suggestion about greater subsequent improvement among patients from the medical unit is more important. Twining and Chapman (1980) show from data published by Garraway and colleagues that there is no difference between stroke and medical unit patients in the proportion who were independent following discharge but dependent 1 year later; but that, of those dependent at discharge, 6% from the stroke unit were independent at follow-up compared with 24% of those from the medical unit. Those patients from the medical unit who became independent had stayed in hospital for a shorter period than other patients in the medical units, and 'we postulate that their full rehabilitations potential had not been realised when they were discharged from hospital' (Garraway *et al.*, 1980*a*, p. 828). A *Lancet* editorial (1981) goes further, suggesting that patients who learnt their independence at home, with their families near them, were more strongly motivated to succeed.

Can we conclude that stroke units confer no advantage? Probably not, because the Edinburgh study does show more rapid improvement in the shorter term for stroke unit patients, which has implications for reducing overall lengths of hospital stay and the fitness of patients on discharge to the 'community'. The study confirms, however, the need to support patients and their families outside hospital and in the longer term. It also raises questions about the appropriateness of focusing exclusively upon functional performance as a measure of outcome. If this is not the only goal of rehabilitation, why was there no assessment of social or family adjustment and emotional well-being? Perhaps the interest, optimism and encouragement in a stroke unit has implications for the way in which patients respond to a stroke, and for their self-concept (which may be more significant to the patient than the ability to be completely independent in self-care). The ambience of the stroke unit may also influence relatives, perhaps making them more alarmed (Vetter, 1980), but perhaps making them more confident about their ability to care after discharge. Murray and colleagues (1982) note that the relatives of stroke unit patients were more likely to describe the ward as 'friendly' and 'relaxed'. The contribution of rehabilitation units to outcomes other than functional performance merits attention.

In Greenwich, patients were not randomly allocated to either the stroke unit or different sorts of therapy; any differences in outcome may therefore be due as much to selection as to effectiveness of the therapy. First, changes in Barthel scores were investigated, again acknowledging that these reflect fairly gross changes in dependency and indicate nothing about the quality of performance. Changes in level of disability are presented in Table 22 for the 'good prospects', since they represent the core group receiving treatment.

None of these differences, suggestive of some benefit from therapy, was statistically significant; nor were there any differences in the proportions of each group who improved or deteriorated. The numbers in each group are small, though, and such analyses take no account of therapy from supporters or nurses. Similar analyses of recovery among patients in the Oxfordshire study (Davies *et al.*, 1989) indicated no advantage to the patients receiving therapy. In Greenwich there was no indication that therapy caused patients to have a more positive attitude to their disability. Use of therapy in the first month was not associated with patients' views, 18 months after the stroke, on the extent or quality of their recovery, expectations for further recovery, hope for the future, or satisfaction with life.

Patients on the stroke unit appeared to improve more than other hospital patients; among patients with moderate or severe disability, those on the stroke unit improved their disability score by an average of 4.8 points, compared with an average of 1.8 for patients elsewhere. Altogether, stroke unit patients improved by 4.1 points on the disability

Table 22. *Changes in patients' disability scores by use of remedial therapy in the first 3 weeks after the stroke*

Use of:	Change from 1 month to 9 months after stroke	Change from 1 month to 18 months after stroke	Change from before stroke to 18 months after stroke
Physiotherapy			
Yes	+2.4 (69)[a]	+2.1 (57)	−4.0 (57)
No	+1.8 (16)	+1.0 (15)	−2.5 (15)
Occupational therapy			
Yes	+2.5 (48)	+2.4 (43)	−4.1 (43)
No	+2.0 (35)	+1.1 (28)	−3.3 (28)

[a] Numbers in brackets are the totals on which scores are based.

index between 1 and 9 months after the stroke compared with an average increase of 1.4 points among patients on other wards. This difference in favour of the stroke unit was particularly clear for patients under 80 years of age. In particular, patients admitted onto the stroke unit within 1 month of the stroke improved more in self-care performance than other hospital patients; between 1 and 9 months their score increased by 2.2 points compared with 0.6 points for patients on other wards. (When only those with moderate or severe disability are considered, the corresponding figures are 3.0 and 1.2.) These differences in disability score were not eroded in the longer term, up to the third interview, unlike the comparative advantage of patients in the randomised trial (Garraway *et al.*, 1980*a*). Possibly the stroke unit patients do better, especially in self-care skills, because they receive more therapy. However, as indicated above, patients who received occupational therapy did not, in general, improve more than those who received none.

It may be that stroke unit patients improved more because their care was both more intensive and better co-ordinated on a ward which encouraged a team approach to rehabilitation. Perhaps also the ward atmosphere was more conducive to patients and supporters developing positive attitudes to rehabilitation. Only 5% of the supporters of patients on the stroke unit thought, 1 month after the stroke, that the patient would make little or no recovery, compared with 37% of the supporters of patients on other wards; and only 5% of patients on the stroke unit felt they would recover little or not at all, compared with 16% of patients on other wards (though this latter difference is not statistically significant). One month after the stroke, patients on the stroke unit were no more or less concerned by the illness than were other patients, nor did morale (assessed in terms of emotional distress) appear to differ from that of patients on other wards. Although, as the next chapter will suggest, patients' attitudes and social integration were important factors related to functional improvement, there were no gross differences between patients on the stroke unit and elsewhere in these aspects. The apparent success in rehabilitation by the stroke unit was not entirely expected (cf. Wade *et al.*, 1985*b*), and it remains difficult to establish what elements of the routine, rehabilitation or ward atmosphere contribute (cf. Garraway *et al.*, 1980*b*).

In considering the value of a stroke unit, it probably should be borne in mind that, unlike the patients in the Edinburgh trial (Garraway *et al.*, 1980*b*), those in Greenwich who went onto the stroke unit in the acute phase stayed in hospital longer. Among patients with severe or very severe disability at 1 month after the stroke, all of those on the stroke unit stayed 12 or more weeks, compared with 58% of other patients.

It was evident thmost of the general practitioners in the health district valued the presence of a stroke unit even if relatively few of their patients were actually treated there. In response to a direct question, 68% of the general practitioners said they thought that a stroke unit conferred advantages for patients, 3% felt there were disadvantages, 6% that there was no difference between the stroke unit and elsewhere, and 23% made some other comment, including:

How long have they had a stroke unit?

Good idea, didn't know of its existence.

Have they got a special stroke unit?

For most of the general practitioners a stroke unit appeared to reflect their preference for a positive, energetic approach to treatment and rehabilitation of patients. Thus some of the advantage was in comparison with unacceptable practice elsewhere:

Patient not regarded as a bloody nuisance. On a general ward the patient is regarded as a pain in the backside. Not geared up.

They are seen as an encumbrance on a medical ward and given a low priority.

Many doctors, though, felt that a stroke unit put the accent on early and intensive rehabilitation:

A team whose minds are directed towards rehabilitation. Therefore, the patient gets physiotherapy regularly without having to vie with other patients for attention.

Article in *BMJ* showed that if you start active physiotherapy early they do better. They improve their function. Initial few days the most important.

There was no unanimity about the psychological benefits of the stroke unit: some doctors held that company of other patients with the same problem was an incentive, or at least better than that of senile patients on geriatric wards; others that it may be depressing for patients to see lots of other strokes, or that patients may be discouraged by seeing people who are worse. Among patients in the study there was no overall difference in measures of emotional distress, isolation, or attitudes to the future between patients who were treated on the stroke unit and elsewhere.

Several of the general practitioners commented that a stroke unit, used as it currently is as an in-patient service, deprives patients of the stimulation, support and skills of people at home. On the other hand it was also argued that a stroke unit has educational benefits:

Family gets a lot of support and are taught how to look after the sick person, and are helped to accept the situation.

It's a shock to the family in the first place. On the stroke unit, the patient can receive intensive care and be educated to manage and accept, and the family can be helped to have him back.

Among the supporters of stroke patients in our study at 9 months after the stroke, there were no differences between those of patients who were or were not treated on the stroke unit in terms of reported satisfaction with contacts with either hospital doctors or nurses. However, 41% of the supporters of patients who had been on the stroke unit reported helpful advice or instruction from a physiotherapist or occupational therapist compared with only 12% of the supporters of patients on other wards. In this respect, at least, the staff on the stroke unit appeared, as in Edinburgh (Murray, *et al.*, 1982), to involve the carers in rehabilitation more usefully.

Attitudes to rehabilitation

There has been very little research into the attitudes of patients and their supporters to the help they receive. In the previous chapter it was shown that many patients had relatively high hopes of the contribution that rehabilitation would make to recovery. At the second interview they were asked about the rehabilitation they had received and several expressed disappointment; some about its mundane content, but others about the lack of rehabilitation they had received.

Patients' descriptions of their therapy emphasise its everyday character; a woman who was discharged home after 2 weeks said she received:

Physiotherapy – they didn't give me any treatment. They just watched me walk down the ward on two days. That was it.

And a man who spent 2 months in hospital graduated through occupational therapy:

Used to be a young girl and we played big games, draughts and so on made out of wood. The O.T. officer now sees me in carpentry, but doesn't bother me very much.

At their second interview, around 9 months after the stroke, several patients commented that really they would have preferred more therapy; for example, two men in their sixties, who, 4 weeks after a stroke, were both severely disabled, said:

[I had] physiotherapy about once or twice a week, which I don't think is enough.

Physiotherapist decided that I would benefit from intensive physiotherapy which was nice of her, but it wasn't actually all that intensive. I decided after two weeks it would be just as good if went in two days a week. They say you should start physiotherapy as soon as possible after the stroke, but down in [a hospital outside the district] I just sat around taking tablets I could have taken at home.

Other patients felt they simply did not have enough therapy for it to be effective. Two women, for example, who were at home a few weeks after the stroke, wondered whether more could not have been done to reduce their 'mild' disability:

I didn't go for long enough to get anything out of it, when they decided they wouldn't do anything more for me. And that seemed right because I was getting better and it seemed to be for people who couldn't move. There should really be something else for people who are getting better or even a lecture to let you know what to do.

Didn't do a lot. I was going to be put in for a lot but it got pushed to one side, so I really didn't do anything. Might have been better if I did.

Patients were not asked systematically about the service they had received, but there were also expressions of satisfaction:

Very useful. Go down, get your dinner, cook it – that's very handy if you've got to come home for that.

Everyday I went down for physiotherapy and they taught me to do things to strengthen my arms. And they got me planting pots and stretching to play a sort of darts. Very nice girls.

The interest of therapists and their positive approach are qualities that appear important to the patients, particularly in the very early stages after the stroke. However, few patients volunteered comments about therapists as sources of information and support. These comments were made by the patients at the second interview when nearly all had been discharged from therapy and when the slow pace of recovery was clear:

I suppose I've been packed up since about February, but I thought at that time they were doing me some good and it came as a bit of a shock. Although it hurt my feelings at the time, on reflection it was reasonable. I think they could see this was going to be a long job and wasn't going anywhere.

This decline in contact, and in pace of improvement, may be one reason why the support and encouragement of therapists was hardly mentioned at the second interview, although this had been commented on in responses made about 4 weeks after the stroke. At the earlier stage the first 50 patients in the study were asked how much the therapists, nurses and doctors gave them support and encouragement; nearly two-thirds of the patients said 'a lot':

Only the therapists. I've only seen the doctor once. He spoke to me.

I haven't done much since I've been here, really. I went to the therapists two or three days ago. They are all very kind in here.

However, this acknowledgement and appreciation of the encouragement given by therapists was tinged with doubt about the real prospects. Many of the patients made comments which reflected their own uncertainties; and more than half of them said they did not know how much the therapists and hospital staff expected them to recover, even though the staff had encouraged them:

They always turn round and say you're alright, but in hospital they never tell you any different.

Do they tell you the truth? 'You'll recover, there's nothing to worry about', they say. But then, they go to the back and they say 'Bad luck on him'.

They're all so bright and breezy – if [improvement in] the hand is possible it [i.e. recovery] would be complete because I have a will to recover. I think they're good here but they've got to be careful what they do. Do I believe, or do I think they are saying sweet things to me?

In these early weeks most patients are hoping for a good recovery; therapists appear to foster and encourage the relatively optimistic expectations that patients have for themselves. In the longer term it appears that the contribution of therapists is judged in terms of their impact on physical recovery, and for many reasons – content, amount, effectiveness – patients were often disappointed.

There appears to be some illusion that therapists make a major contribution as advisers or supporters to the patient's family. However, reports from supporters of help from therapists were relatively uncommon. At the first interview only 1 in 10 supporters identified a physiotherapist or an occupational therapist as a source of advice or information about how they could help the stroke patient. The wife of a man in his sixties with severe physical and communication impairment reported help from the therapists:

They've told us to talk to him. Sit the left-side of him, massage his legs when we sit with him.

Another wife commented on support from both physiotherapy and occupational therapy:

I used to watch him have his therapy. I know there are some things I can do to help him. It's helped a lot.

And one woman mentioned help from a domiciliary physiotherapist:

Physiotherapist showed me how to exercise his legs and toes. I don't mind at all.

A small number of these early contacts with therapists were linked to the patient's discharge. The husband of a woman with severe disability, but who came home after 2 weeks in hospital, reported that the occupational therapist:

Came here and they put boards under the mattress and she had prescribed a special chair for her. I feel quite happy; but I was really surprised when she was discharged. The O.T. said she'd like to come home with us to see if there was anything we needed. They were very helpful, but they said can you have her home tomorrow. I thought they could have been more reasonable in helping her to walk a bit more or made sure I could manage with her.

In several cases the communication between supporter and therapist appeared to be slight in content:

Physiotherapist phoned and said he ought to have a bed downstairs, but he won't agree.

Physiotherapist? I saw her putting him through his paces, that's all.

Perhaps because these contacts were relatively short-lived and uneventful, few were recalled when supporters were asked 8 months later about contacts with therapists since the stroke. Altogether, only 22% of supporters said they had seen a physiotherapist or occupational therapist since the stroke, although nearly three-quarters of these contacts were described as helpful. Nearly half of these helpful contacts were recalled by the supporters of patients who had spent some time on the stroke unit. They were made up of advice on movement of the patient and on therapy at home; and of contacts made by the occupational therapist to check facilities in the patient's home:

Just advice on how to transfer her from bed to the wheelchair; she's been very helpful.

[Advice] that they shouldn't use an exercising thing for their hand – like a rubber ball – because it's very hard work and unnatural. They should keep their fingers moving without a ball.

O.T. came and saw what else was needed. They had bars put up and made gadgets for her.

These helpful contacts with the physiotherapist or occupational therapist were reported by more of the spouses of stroke patients (27%) than by other supporters, only 10% of whom reported contact that provided helpful advice or instruction. The main characteristic associated with supporters' reports of helpful advice was, however, the severity of the patient's disability 1 month after the stroke: nearly half (48%) of the supporters of patients with severe disability said they had received helpful advice, but none of the supporters of patients with very severe disability said this, and only 4% of the supporters of patients who were classified as having moderate or mild disability recalled helpful contact with a physiotherapist or occupational therapist.

If physical therapists are going to make the most of their potential for improving the lives of stroke patients and their families, they must involve the supporters. It is a delusion to believe that professionals can fill all the gaps, or that they can be sensitive to the needs and aspirations of patients in the way most supporters can. Considering that, at the time of the stroke, half the supporters lived at home with the patient, their involvement in rehabilitation appears to be slight. This is important not only because a reservoir of 'natural helpers' is untapped but because the knowledge and skills of supporters are not being developed – at least not by the therapists.

Therapy for speech-impaired patients

In the first interview, about 4 weeks after the stroke, 25% of patients were classified as having some problem with speech, and a further 11% were assessed as having a major problem. Altogether 22% of patients received some help from a speech therapist in the first few weeks: that comprised 8% of patients who were defined as having no speech problem (they may have recovered or had some other difficulty, with comprehension or swallowing for example), 50% of patients with some problem, and 56% of those with a major problem. Male patients with a speech problem appeared to be more likely to receive help: of those patients with a major problem, 77% of the men but only 29% of the women patients received speech therapy. This curious difference is related in part to the fact that the women were older: of people aged 75 or over with a speech problem only 34% received speech therapy compared with 77% of younger patients. This may be because the limited resources for speech therapy are not directed to cover the geriatric wards; among patients with a speech problem only 33% of those on geriatric wards had speech therapy compared with 63% of these patients in general medical beds. Again, where the patient is in the hospital affects the treatment received. The degree of physical disability of a patient with speech problems was not generally associated with whether or not that patient saw a speech therapist.

Among patients who survived to the second interview at around 9 months after the stroke, a quarter of those who began speech therapy in the first month were still receiving it. Only two patients began speech therapy after the first interview and all the patients who were having speech therapy over the longer term were at home.

The classification of speech problems into 'none', 'some' and 'major' is not based upon a sophisticated formal examination and is clearly not sensitive to minor changes. This classification did not reveal any improvement in the speech of patients receiving therapy beyond that achieved by patients in the same category who did not receive therapy; the outcome was surprisingly in the opposite direction: of the patients whose expression was classified as 'some problem' at the first interview, 8% of those who had speech therapy, but 43% of those who did not, were classified as 'no problem' at the second interview. Possibly, people were being treated who had little potential for recovery. However, the crude measurement employed in this study does not form the basis for a significant contribution to the debate about the effectiveness of speech therapy (David *et al.*, 1982; Lincoln *et al.*, 1984).

The evidence of recovery of speech is not strong: only 18% of the patients with a speech problem at the first interview were classified as having 'no problem' 18 months later. More extensive research on the natural history of aphasia has similarly found a high correlation between early and later scores, Wade and colleagues reporting that only 18% of patients who were aphasic at 3 weeks after a stroke recovered to 'normal' by 6 months (Wade *et al.*, 1986*a*). But major changes in speech are not expected; rather the aim of therapy is to facilitate 'communication' in different ways and to improve the patient's self-image. There were, however, no differences in general satisfaction in favour of speech-impaired patients who had therapy; again it was the group of patients who initially had a speech problem but who did not have speech therapy who felt they had recovered better – three-quarters of them said they had recovered 'a lot' compared with only a quarter of the patients who had speech therapy. Patients who had speech therapy were no more or less likely than others with speech problems to return to their pre-stroke level of social activities or family contacts.

Patients who were given speech therapy may have had different speech problems to the older patients who did not have treatment. Those who received the treatment may or may not have improved their communication. Certainly, many of those having speech therapy found it enjoyable or felt it was useful, although they said relatively little about this. A few patients were more critical and seemed to find the exercise unrewarding. A woman whose only problem was with speech felt:

It was very childish – What's that? What's that? I felt uncomfortable, but I suppose she had to do it. I was still slurring a little. She was ever so pleased.

In the longer term, treatment was often in a group rather than one-to-one therapy:

It's a self-help group now. We go in, we do our own thing. Speech therapist says that they can't hear me, the other people, when I talk. So I write my name and a sentence on the board. I write 'The Child of a New Age' and they see how many words they can get out of that. All the patients who've freshly had a stroke, the speech therapists see to them on the wards and we go downstairs to do our self-help group. Sometimes I think it's a waste of time, but we have a laugh. Whenever I've been depressed I think I'll go, it will be a break. There's always something to laugh about or talk about.

It is particularly for speech-impaired patients that involvement of relatives appears to be useful for the patients themselves (David *et al.*, 1982), and probably necessary to prevent difficulties for carers (Kinsella and Duffy, 1979). Lincoln and colleagues (1984) have concluded that speech therapists could be more effective if they placed more emphasis on giving advice to relatives on how to cope with problems in communication.

All supporters were asked at the second interview whether they had had any contact with a speech therapist since the patient's stroke. Only 7 supporters (21% of the supporters of patients who had a speech problem

4 weeks after the stroke) said they had, of whom 5 reported that the contact had been helpful. On this basis, the contribution of speech therapists to helping supporters directly and, through them, to reducing the patient's handicap, is marginal. Yet results from this study, detailed in Chapter 7, suggest that speech-impaired patients and their supporters have a particular need for support to prevent deterioration in close relationships.

Ambitions for the future

The patients in Greenwich were predominantly working-class. This may account in part for the generally modest aspirations that patients had 1 month after the stroke. All the patients were asked in this first interview what, for them, would be the most important thing to achieve or do again. Their answers gave the impression that, on the one hand, they did not think about this a lot and, on the other hand, that if the future was about getting back to normal it depended upon the single ability of being able to walk:

What I'd like to do most of all? Walk like I always used to. Very fond of a walk on Sunday; would like to do that again.

To be able to walk, even with the aid of a stick.

To be able to walk is to be able to do things – to go in the garden, to the pub, to the church, or take the dogs in the park. For many of the women, returning to normal life meant getting back to housework and shopping; for example, two women who, before the stroke, had done everything for themselves symbolised their return to normal life in domestic terms:

Walk out and catch the bus and go to Woolwich and do my shopping.

Get on my feet and go out and do my shopping and come home and do my work as I've always been doing.

Not surprisingly, people want to retain their independence and resist becoming a burden to others:

Just to be able to do my bit, meet my family and not be a burden to anybody.

Only 3 patients said that returning to paid work was the most important thing. This was not surprising given the small number employed before the stroke.

Sadly 1 in 8 of the patients who answered this question (which therefore excludes the most seriously ill) could see nothing to aim for. One man, who before the stroke had been caring for his handicapped wife, said:

That's another funny question; there isn't anything to look forward to now.

Several other patients were more fatalistic. One man who died 3 weeks later, said:

Don't think of anything like that. My time is up and that's the end of it.

And a woman who had returned home from hospital but who did not expect to recover viewed the future in terms of:

Going in my coffin . . . I can't drink, I can't eat, I can't smoke, I can't make love; all I can do is sit here.

Other than returning as fast as possible to life before the stroke, patients had few specific plans or aspirations. Their ambitions were generally modest:

I've got no ambition to do anything other than live. I've no business. All I want to do is make sure I've no debts.

and they were flexible:

I've got plenty of dreams and ideas, but none are so important that it would be the end of the world. I'm prepared to settle for what I can get.

Perhaps this capacity to live with modest aspirations and to accommodate ambition to prevailing circumstances enabled many patients to maintain an optimistic outlook in the face of serious disability. At the interview 4 weeks after the stroke two-thirds of the patients described themselves as hopeful about the future, 9% were not very hopeful and 23% were uncertain. Although these attitudes were not strongly associated with level of disability, 22% of patients with severe or very severe disability were not very hopeful compared with only 7% of less disabled patients.

Several patients were uncertain or pessimistic about the future because of issues other than the stroke, such as family problems, housing and other illness, but health and recovery from the stroke appeared, unsurprisingly, to be the main issue. For a few patients, uncertainty about the future was strongly related to concerns about their treatment since the stroke. Patients were uncertain because:

I know nothing you see. I mean they don't really tell you how you are doing. All they said is 'Oh, you've improved', which is a load of old codswallop.

I don't think anyone coming round here every five weeks to ask you if you'll wiggle your little finger is any use. And probably next time you come to see me I shall be nearer a human cabbage than I am now. Amen. I'll just be a geriatric old sod who doesn't know what he's doing.

However, it was also apparent that relatively few patients had begun to think much about the future; they were often bewildered and preoccupied by present problems. One housebound woman expressed the dilemma as:

I'm worried about the future, I'm worried about today. You can't plan the future.

The supporters appeared to be somewhat less hopeful about the future than patients: 14% of them described their view of the future as not very hopeful, 40% were uncertain and only 46% said they were hopeful.

Male supporters appeared to be more optimistic than women (58% of men were hopeful about the patient's future compared with 41% of women); and working-class supporters were more likely to describe themselves as hopeful, 58% of them saying this compared with only 29% of supporters who were categorised as middle-class. The supporter's age was not an important factor, but supporters of older patients were less hopeful. The proportion of supporters who described themselves as hopeful fell from 62% of the supporters of patients aged 60–64, to only 28% of the supporters of patients aged 80 and over.

Worries about the future

In these early weeks after the stroke, services are being organised for rehabilitation and to prepare patients for a future in the community. The anxieties and problems of patients and their families are relevant to all staff who hope to help in making realistic preparations and providing timely, useful advice. However, the concerns and perspectives of patients appear to be different from those of their carers. Carers are already thinking about how the patient will cope outside hospital (and, therefore, how they themselves will cope), while many patients seem likely to consider advice about the longer term to be inappropriate. Both patients and their supporters were asked at 1 month after the stroke what their main worries were about the future for the patient. A majority of the patients replied that they had no major worries about the future; a perspective which was shared by only 1 in 8 of their supporters. Occasionally there seemed to be a particularly good reason for the patient to view the future with equanimity; a woman who needed a wheelchair to get about, but who lived with her husband in sheltered housing, replied:

Well, I don't let anything worry me about it, because I'm in a lovely place to be looked after and an easily run flat.

Her husband was more cautious:

The main worry is getting about; but we don't know until she gets home anyway.

The future is, of course, precarious; in this case the return home was successful but the patient's husband died just a few weeks later.

In most cases where the patients felt there were no worries, their supporters disagreed. Few patients seemed to 'deny' completely that there would be difficulties; rather they viewed them as not important or 'major' worries. Commonly, the supporters were concerned about housing, about where and with whom the patient was going to live, whereas the patient was not. A man in his mid-seventies who lived in a boarding house said there were no worries, but his friend and landlady for 20 years was:

Trying to get him somewhere to go when he comes out of hospital. He's got to go into a nursing home. He thinks he's coming home but I doubt it. It would mean having someone here all day. We want to get him to a nursing home first; he's quite prepared to pay.

Another man who was unable to walk and lived on the fourth floor of a block of council flats with no lift, said he had no worries, possibly because he felt leaving hospital was still in the distant future. But his sister was concerned:

I couldn't have him here because of the stairs. Where will he live?

Supporters also appeared to be more concerned about the social and psychological well-being of patients. A man with mild disability who lived alone at home said, regarding main worries, 'I don't have any, not really'. But his daughter was concerned:

My main worry is that he'll be unhappy. I'm worried about him getting very depressed. He's nearly blind now and he can't walk out in the High Street every day. He has no friends. He's a loner. He's getting a bit irritable now.

This concern about the patient's mental state was mentioned by a quarter of the supporters, even of patients who appeared to have adopted the lowest-key coping strategies. One man who spent only a few weeks in hospital reflected that:

I don't sit there and fret. I'm accepting it as it comes, but I'm fairly philosophical about the whole thing.

His wife, however, saw another side to his character, which was often expressed by supporters:

We can cope providing he doesn't get too frustrated. I think that will be the biggest bugbear really.

In practice, 'frustration' was to prove a major problem for both patient and supporter.

In other cases the patients foresaw no main worries at least in part because, following the stroke, they were less well oriented and had less insight into problems. One woman, who moved to her son's home, felt she had no worries about the future. In the circumstances this was true, but her daughter-in-law thought the patient would have problems coping:

Mentally, I think. As far as her looking after herself is concerned, I think this is the biggest thing. And she couldn't cope with handling hot things. I'm afraid she would scald herself. She's very confused mentally.

On the whole it seems that, at this stage after the stroke, patients found it difficult to envisage a plan for the future, particularly from their hospital bed. Their priorities were relatively short term: to improve their walking, get home and then see how things were. The patients' main worries were usually not articulated in the interviews, nor it appeared did patients themselves dwell on or make these anxieties too explicit. Their lack of worries about the future was complemented by the supporters, few of whom did not have some major concern, particularly about housing and the patient's mental state. At this stage after the stroke the illness was more threatening to many of the supporters than it was to the patients.

SUMMARY

There has been little systematic information about the attitudes and daily experience of stroke patients in hospital. In this study about two-thirds of the patients recalled some particularly positive aspect of life in hospital, most commonly that the staff, especially the nurses, had been caring and kind. The problem about being in hospital that appeared to cause most distress also referred to nurses: it was the difficulty of attracting their attention, especially for the toilet and especially at night. Less than half of all patients identified something about their experience in hospital which especially upset them.

Rehabilitation Altogether four-fifths of the patients received some physiotherapy in the first month, and two-fifths had occupational therapy. The proportion who received therapy was greater among patients who had spent all of the acute phase in hospital, and did not vary with hospital or ward, except that stroke unit patients were more likely to have had occupational therapy. Physiotherapy tended to be given most to patients with moderate or severe disability; occupational therapy was given when patients were less disabled and was much less likely to go to patients who were incontinent. There was no evidence of targeting occupational therapy to patients with perceptual or sensory difficulties. The pattern of use of therapy is established within the first weeks after the stroke. In general, patients who received rehabilitation differed little in their ability to perform activities of daily living from those who did not. This would be important if it could be shown that patients who have therapy benefit from it; the results from previous research are inconclusive. In this study, which was not, of course, a controlled trial, there were some indications that patients who had therapy made more improvement in their independence in activities of daily living, but they were no more likely in the long term to report a better quality of life.

Patients on the stroke unit, especially those under 80 years of age, appeared to improve more than other hospital patients. This apparent advantage to stroke unit patients was not eroded during the course of the research, but it was difficult to identify a good reason for the difference. However, patients in Greenwich who went onto the stroke unit in the first weeks stayed in hospital longer. Two-thirds of the general practitioners in Greenwich thought that the stroke unit conferred advantages for patients.

In the early stages many patients expressed their appreciation for the support given by therapists but, as physical recovery waned, there was often disappointment – about the content, frequency or effectiveness of the rehabilitation. Supporters reported relatively little contact with therapists; altogether only 22% said they had seen a physiotherapist or occupational therapist in the 9 months after the stroke, although three-quarters of these contacts were described as helpful. Rehabilitation staff on the stroke unit appeared to involve supporters more usefully in rehabilitation. Helpful contacts with therapists were reported most often by the spouses of stroke patients, and predominantly by the supporters of patients who had severe disability.

About half the patients with a speech impairment received speech therapy; and patients on general medical rather than geriatric wards were more likely to receive this. Many appeared to feel it had been useful, even though various assessments indicated no advantage to the group who had received therapy. There was little involvement of supporters in speech therapy, although the social and family relationships of speech-impaired patients were particularly likely to deteriorate.

Attitudes to the future   The attitudes of patients were clearly associated with expectations for recovery, particularly regaining the ability to walk. Perhaps because their aspirations were different, patients and supporters classified as working-class appeared to have a more positive outlook.

Patients and their supporters appeared to have different concerns at 1 month after the stroke, with supporters thinking more about the future, especially about housing and the patient's mental health. They had, therefore, rather different needs for information.

CHAPTER FIVE

Survival, physical disability and health

Survival

The literature on survival following stroke (see Chapter 1) indicates strongly that the core group of deaths occur in the first few weeks after the stroke. Nevertheless, there appears to be a relatively high mortality rate throughout the year after stroke, and studies of more disabled samples of patients (Brocklehurst *et al.*, 1978*a*; Stevens and Ambler, 1982) – as this one is – suggest that perhaps one-third of the patients will die between 1 and 12 months after the stroke. The figures in Table 23 show that altogether 36% of patients died before the end of the first year, and that most of these were deaths before 3 months after the stroke. The proportion of patients who died and, in particular, the proportion who died between 1 and 3 months after the stroke was, as found in other studies, clearly related to the severity of the patient's disability.

Among the various clinical assessments, the absence of normal sitting balance appears to be a particularly strong predictor of early death; 51% of those with abnormal sitting balance died between 1 and 3 months after the stroke, compared with 11% of patients who were able to maintain an upright sitting position. The significance of perceptual and sensory deficits has been identified in recent hospital-based studies (Henley *et al.*, 1985; Fullerton *et al.*, 1986). Among the Greenwich patients, those with major proprioceptive loss (in both wrist and finger) were less likely to survive to 1 year after the stroke than other patients who could be tested (53% did compared with 80% of others); and the proportion who survived to 1 year was 76% among patients with 'normal' sensation but only 60% for patients with reduced or no sensation in the affected hand.

However, it is the patients who cannot be tested like this who are most likely to die: only 28% of the patients who could not follow the test for proprioceptive loss were alive 1 year after the stroke. These patients who

Table 23. *Patients' severity of disability 1 month after stroke related to survival: proportion surviving for different periods*

Survival after stroke (months)	Barthel rating at 1 month					
	Very severe (%)	Severe (%)	Moderate (%)	Mild (%)	Normal (%)	All patients (%)
1 to <3	58	23	8	10	0	22
3 to <6	10	10	15	2	0	8
6 to <9	6	0	8	2	0	3
9 to <12	3	8	0	0	0	3
12 or more	23	59	69	86	100	64
No. of patients (=100%)	31	52	26	42	15	166

could not be tested were too ill or confused or their communication too impaired to participate. Isaacs and Marks (1973) suggested that tests of cognitive function should be part of the clinical examination of stroke patients. This deficit was clearly associated with the outcome for patients in Greenwich, for among those scoring 5 or more on the Walkey (orientation) test 80% were alive 1 year after the stroke, compared with 41% of those who scored 3 or less, and only 11% of the patients who were unable to respond to the questions in the test. These results are among the clearest predictors of survival. However, as Sheikh and colleagues (1983) note, so many characteristics of the stroke are related to each other and to the severity of disability that it is difficult to identify which factors make important independent contributions to the outcome.

Patients with severe, moderate or mild disability have been discussed as 'good prospects' for survival (in Chapter 4). Among these patients there were some differences between those who did and did not survive for a year after the stroke. The differentiating characteristics are shown in Table 24. Survival after the first month, like survival of the acute episode (Wade *et al.*, 1984), is lower among patients who are incontinent. Altogether, only 42% of the patients who were catheterised at the time of the first interview at 4 weeks after the stroke survived to 1 year after the stroke; and 53% of them died between 1 and 6 months after the stroke.

The patient's mental state is a relatively neglected variable in the analyses of case-fatality, although among patients with good prospects those whose cognition was moderately or severely impaired were much less likely to survive to 1 year after the stroke; and 48% of these patients (scoring 0–4 on the Walkey test) died between 1 and 6 months after the

Table 24. *Some characteristics of the patient related to survival in patients with 'good prospects'*

Characteristics at 1 month after the stroke	Proportion alive 1 year after the stroke	
Incontinence of:		
Urine		
No	80%	(79)[a]
Yes	54%	(41)
Faeces		
No	75%	(102)
Yes	50%	(18)
Walkey score:		
5–8 (better)	78%	(93)
0–4 (worse)	44%	(25)
Emotional score:		
0–5 (better)	82%	(84)
6–9 (worse)	47%	(19)
Social isolation score:		
0–3 (better)	81%	(88)
4–5 (worse)	45%	(11)
Sex:		
Female	87%	(68)
Male	50%	(52)

[a] Figures in brackets are the numbers on which percentages are based.

stroke. This is probably associated with impaired consciousness during the acute phase, which is a well-established factor associated with early death (Aho *et al.*, 1980). Two-thirds of the patients with cognitive deficits were unable to respond to items on the Nottingham Health Profile; however, the patients whose answers indicated high levels of emotional distress or feelings of social isolation had relatively poor prognoses for survival. The significance of the patient's mood state for outcome has been registered elsewhere (Henley *et al.*, 1985) and would seem to merit further investigation. The psychological response to stroke, whether caused by brain damage or feelings of disadvantage, may be reflected in perceptions of hopelessness and helplessness (Abramson *et al.*, 1978).

Among the patients who were good prospects 83% of those who described themselves as hopeful about the future were alive 1 year after the stroke compared with 66% of those who said they were not hopeful, or were uncertain. Again, though, only 41% of these patients who were unable to respond to this question survived to a year after the stroke. This last group consists principally of patients who were disoriented, but also includes some with a communication deficit. Among patients with good prospects whose speech could be assessed, only 57% of those with a speech problem survived for a year compared with 76% of patients without difficulty in expressing themselves. This may reflect the extent of the brain lesion, or somehow relate to the patient's mood and attitudes to the stroke.

A comparison of these results with those from other studies is of dubious value since few studies have looked at subsequent mortality among people who survived the acute episode. However, Henley and colleagues (1985) began with patients alive 2 weeks after the stroke and looked at deaths over the next year. They reported that women were more likely to die, which is the opposite of the finding among patients in this study (see Table 24). Henley and colleagues (1985) found an increasing death rate among older patients. In our study there is no association between survival and age of patient among the good prospects but, altogether, the proportion of patients who survived until a year after the stroke fell from 81% of those aged 60–64 at the time of the stroke to only 45% of patients aged 85 or more. Age is therefore a dominant parameter for survival, but in this study it is no longer important after controlling for severity of the disability. There was some indication that patients with severe disability at 1 month after the stroke survived longer if they had been admitted to the stroke unit: 71% of them were still alive 1 year after the stroke compared with only 38% of severely disabled patients who were on other hospital wards.

Physical disability

This section will concentrate on changes over the course of the study in the mobility, self-care and disability of patients, and will look at the condition of their lives in the longer term. Few patients died between the second and third interviews (at 9 and 18 months after the stroke, respectively), and so most analyses of change and recovery will focus on patients seen at all three stages after the stroke.

Physical disability as an outcome of stroke should be distinguished from functional improvement and return to normal. It is quite possible, for example, for a patient to improve significantly after a stroke but nevertheless to be disabled and unable to perform activities that were possible before the stroke. The views of patients and their supporters about these three aspects of recovery may differ from each other and also fail to reflect the changes measured by the researcher.

A recurring, but somewhat paradoxical finding is that patients who achieve the greatest functional improvement following the stroke are also

Table 25. *Patients' disability at 1 month related to functional*
improvement by third interview at 18 months

Change in disability score	Barthel rating at 1 month				
	Severe (9 or less) (%)	Moderate (10–14) (%)	Mild (15–19) (%)	Normal (20) (%)	All patients (%)
+5 or more	44	27	0	0	20
+3 or 4	13	13	24	0	15
+1 or 2	31	13	46	0	29
0	6	0	9	85	17
−1 or less	6	47	21	15	19
No. of patients (=100%)	32	15	33	13	93
Average change	+3.5	+1.0	+0.7	−0.2	+1.6

the most disabled in the longer term. For example, among patients who improved by 5 or more points on the disability score, only 6% were classified as normal on the Barthel index at the third interview. The corresponding proportion for patients who improved by 1 to 4 points is 27%, while 56% of patients whose score was the same at 4 weeks and 18 months after the stroke were noted as normal, or independent in activities of daily living. The explanation of this paradox is, of course, that patients with greater initial disability have more scope for measurable improvement. This is shown in Table 25, which also indicates that most of the severely disabled patients who survive will improve.

The extent of recovery after stroke has generally been measured in terms of 'outcome'. Several studies (e.g. Wade *et al.*, 1983; Henley *et al.*, 1985) have sought to identify factors which influence outcome in relation to physical disability. All authors have pointed to disability shortly after the stroke as a very important influence. So, as Table 26 shows, most patients remained in the same disability category from first to third interviews or improved by one category. There is, again, considerable improvement seen for some patients classified at the first interview as severely or moderately disabled.

Before the stroke most patients were independent in their activities of daily living and three-quarters were classified as having little or no disability. For these patients their disability score at the third interview is a measure of the extent of change in their functional performance.

Table 26. *Patients' disability at 1 month after the stroke related to that at 18 months*

Barthel rating at 18 months after the stroke	Barthel rating at 1 month				
	Severe (9 or less) (%)	Moderate (10–14) (%)	Mild (15–19) (%)	Normal (20) (%)	All patients (%)
Severe	37	20	3	0	17
Moderate	38	33	6	0	20
Mild	25	40	58	31	40
Normal	0	7	33	69	23
No. of patients (=100%)	32	15	33	13	93

However, disability outcome is an inadequate indicator of change in physical performance for about one-quarter of the survivors to the third interview. In particular, it is likely to underestimate the extent of return to the level of functioning before the stroke among older patients who had more previous disability. For example, 9% of patients who were severely disabled at 1 month after the stroke returned to or improved on their level of performance of activities of daily living that existed before the stroke. This is shown in Table 27, which presents the extent to which patients returned to the level of functioning they had before the stroke. Altogether, by 18 months after the stroke 1 patient in 3 had returned to the same level of (or lack of) disability that existed before the stroke.

The average fall in the disability score was about 3 points from before the stroke to 18 months later. This is reflected in Table 28, which shows large declines following the stroke in the proportion of patients who were independent in the activities that were asked about (most of which are included in the disability rating). Eighteen months after the stroke three-quarters of the patients were dependent in some activity measured for the disability rating. Only 16% of patients who had limb weakness at 1 month after the stroke had none at 18 months. The side of weakness at 1 month after the stroke was not associated with severity of disability in the longer term. Nor were most of the sociodemographic variables – sex, social class, marital status, household size or composition – related to disability at 18 months after the stroke. Only the patient's age was related in any significant way; and even then the only statistically significant trend was a decline with age in the proportion of patients classified as normal. In several other studies (Isaacs and Marks, 1973; Wade *et al.*, 1983; Henley

Table 27. *Patient's disability at 1 month after the stroke related to the extent of their return to pre-stroke performance of activities of daily living*

Compared with before the stroke, disability score at 18 months after stroke is:	Barthel rating at 1 month				
	Severe (9 or less) (%)	Moderate (10–14) (%)	Mild (15–19) (%)	Normal (20) (%)	All patients (%)
Same or better	9	13	52	85	36
− 1 to 4 points	31	47	36	15	33
− 5 to 8 points	29	13	6	0	14
− 9 or more points	31	27	6	0	17
No. of patients (= 100%)	32	15	33	13	93

Table 28. *Changes with time in the proportions of patients[a] who were independent in activities of daily living*

	Before stroke (%)	1 month after (%)	9 months after (%)	18 months after (%)
Mobility				
Bed unaided	96	58	85	82
Chair unaided	98	70	90	84
Outside 50 + yards unaided	71	16	40	38
Up 5 + stairs unaided	81	24	44	42
Down 5 + stairs unaided	80	24	45	42
Drives car	11	–	1	3
Uses bus or train unaccompanied	49	–	20	18
Self-care				
Feeds self without help	95	61	61	58
Dresses without help	89	48	62	56
Grooms self without help	96	73	87	85
Washes body without help	80	30	42	32
Uses lavatory without help	94	58	84	80
Cuts own toenails	44	N/A[b]	22	13

[a] These were patients who were seen at all three interviews: $n = 93$.
[b] N/A, not asked.

Table 29. *Severity of disability of patients[a] 1 month after the stroke related to average disability scores*

Average disability score	Barthel rating at 1 month				
	Severe (9 or less)	Moderate (10–14)	Mild (15–19)	Normal (20)	All
Before stroke	14	14	15	16	15
1 month after stroke	4	9	13	16	10
9 months after stroke	8	12	14	16	12
18 months after stroke	8	10	14	16	11
No. of patients	32	15	33	13	93

[a] These were patients seen at all three interviews: $n = 93$.

et al., 1985) older patients have generally been more dependent. In Greenwich the differences associated with age are less marked, probably because only patients aged 60 and over were entered into the study.

It will be seen in Chapter 8 that a return to pre-stroke performance levels is important to patients and their supporters in their assessment of recovery. From the perspective of doctors and rehabilitation personnel 'functional improvement' is likely to be of particular interest. These two changes are, of course, related to each other ($r = 0.23$), and the discussion of factors influencing change in physical disability focuses on functional improvement.

Functional improvement

The scale of change in measured disability is presented in Table 29, which shows the average disability scores (out of a possible 16) at the various points before and after the stroke. It is clear from this that improvements in functional performance are seen mainly in the severely disabled and, to a lesser extent, moderately disabled groups, but nearly all patients make some physical recovery in the early months (see also Wade and Langton-Hewer, 1987*a*). There was little measured change in performance of the different activities between 9 and 18 months after the stroke; the small decline, principally among people with moderate disability, is mainly due to some loss in the performance of self-care activities. This later loss in performance was more likely among older patients: the proportion of patients whose disability score declined between the second and third

Table 30. *Functional improvement between 1 and 9 months after the stroke for patients with moderate or severe disability*

	Average increase in disability score
Age at stroke:	
60–79	4.0 (40)[a]
80 or more	1.8 (19)
Score on emotional distress at 1 month:	
0–3	4.7 (30)
4 or more	1.9 (18)
Score on social isolation scale at 1 month:	
0	5.4 (16)
1 or more	2.8 (32)

[a] Figures in brackets are the numbers on which the averages are based.

interviews increased from 8% among patients aged 60–69, to 43% of patients aged 80 and over.

The pattern of functional improvement is dominated by the severity of disability 1 month after the stroke. When analysis is confined to the patients making most improvement, i.e. those with moderate or severe disability, then three main variables, in addition to treatment on the stroke unit (see Chapter 4), were associated with the extent of improvement. The relationship between functional improvement and age, emotional distress and social isolation is shown in Table 30. Among all patients age was not a significant factor related to improvement between 1 and 9 months after the stroke, but people aged 80 or over with moderate or severe disability improved less than younger patients with similar levels of physical disability. In the longer term it was found that patients aged 80 and over generally made less progress: altogether, between the first and third interviews, the average disability score of patients aged 80 and over did not change, while younger patients improved on average by 2.1 points. Older people suffer with other chronic illnesses and multiple pathology: it seems likely that they have less physical capacity to develop and maintain their recovery.

When patients were seen first many of their feelings about themselves, their response to stroke, and their recovery – social isolation, stigma, expectations for recovery and views on how much they could help their own recovery (although not others such as emotional distress or hope for the future) – were related to their level of disability. These relationships were consistently that the more disabled patients had more negative attitudes. Since the more disabled patients made more functional improvement it could have been expected that some of these attitudes would be inversely related to change in disability scores between the first and second interviews. However, when all patients are considered only higher levels of 'emotional distress' were associated with lower levels of functional improvement.

When patients with moderate or severe disability are considered then those with lower levels of emotional distress and those who reported no feelings of social isolation did better. In both cases the figures presented in Table 30 are based upon arbitrary divisions in the scores, but in both cases the correlations with functional improvement were highly significant: for emotional distress the coefficient is -0.36, and for social isolation it is -0.38. In another London study (Henley *et al.*, 1985) assessments of the patient's mood were significant predictors of outcome. It is not clear whether mood influences improvement through affecting attitudes to treatment, or more generally through affecting inclination to perform certain activities, or whether there is some other reason. Possibly, emotionally distressed patients are so preoccupied and introspective that they lose interest in recovery; certainly patients who were more emotionally distressed were less likely to feel they could help themselves to recover ($r = -0.47$). There appears to be some support for this suggestion in analysis of some questions which were not part of the assessment of emotional distress. The figures in Table 31 show that, among patients with moderate or severe disability, those who agreed that they had lost interest in things or who felt frustrated with their situation made less improvement.

Several authors (e.g. Litman, 1962) have included feelings of anger or bitterness among the positive mental resources of patients. Andrews and Stewart (1979) note that patients who were reported by their chief carers to have a positive (angry, anxious) attitude to stroke achieved their potential at home better than those with negative (withdrawn, apathetic) attitudes. However, as Table 32 shows, anger was part of a set of 'negative' attitudes among these patients in Greenwich. Feeling angry at their condition was not in general associated with functional improvement, nor significantly with deterioration.

The contribution of psychosocial factors to recovery is not limited to the influences of the patient's feelings following the stroke; it appears, at least in some respects, that patients who were less socially integrated before the stroke did less well (see Table 31). In other respects, for

Table 31. *Specific psychosocial factors related to functional improvement of patients[a] between 1 and 9 months after the stroke*

	Average improvement in disability score
Statements with which patients agreed or disagreed 1 month after stroke:	
I have lost interest in things	
Agree	1.1 (9)[b]
Disagree	4.3 (38)
I feel frustrated with my situation	
Agree	2.5 (24)
Disagree	4.8 (24)
Social integration of the patient 1 month after stroke:	
Agrees with any 'stigma' item	
Yes	1.6 (13)
No	4.4 (35)
Number of close friends	
3 or less	3.0 (32)
4 or more	4.8 (15)
Member of club, group or association	
Yes	3.2 (40)
No	5.5 (10)

[a]Only patients with moderate or severe disability.
[b]Figures in brackets are the numbers on which the average scores are based.

Table 32. *Patients' attitudes associated with feeling angry about the stroke*

	Feel angry that the illness happened to them	
	Yes	No
Average score for:		
Emotional distress	4.26	2.37
Social isolation	1.83	0.87
Proportion:		
Lost interest in things	40%	18%
Feel frustrated with situation	62%	39%
No. of patients (= 100%)	53	71

example marital status and household size, there were no differences in functional improvement following the stroke. Neither widowed patients nor those living alone expressed more feelings of social isolation than others.

The mechanism through which social integration influences functional improvement is a matter for conjecture. In this study social isolation was not related to either the patient's age or disability before the stroke. In earlier studies Litman (1962) and Hyman (1972) reported a relationship between measures of social involvement (social participation, social isolation) and response to rehabilitation. However, among the severely or moderately disabled patients in Greenwich who had rehabilitation (occupational therapy or physiotherapy) there was no significant difference in functional improvement between patients who did and did not report any feelings of social isolation. (Nor did rehabilitation appear to have a significant impact on functional improvement.) The mechanisms by which psychosocial factors influence functional improvement may, therefore, be more general. Previous authors, in common with many practitioners, have ascribed the link in the process to patient 'motivation'. Insofar as this was assessed in the Greenwich study the patients who felt at all isolated were more likely to say they had lost interest in things; 41% said this compared with only 9% of patients who had no score on the measure of social isolation. The question is, what might account for this loss of interest or motivation?

Social factors appear to be related to functional improvement mainly through social and community activities, rather than marital or domestic relationships. Perhaps patients with less community involvement before the stroke feel there is less to return to or less that it is worth while working for. Perhaps also they see themselves as having less need to improve functional performance in order to be able to return to the activities they enjoyed before the stroke. Patients who reported social isolation at the first interview had lower levels of social activities before the stroke: they scored an average of 12.6 points compared with 14.2 points for those patients who reported no feelings of social isolation. Following the stroke, among patients with initially moderate or severe disability there was no difference related to feelings of social isolation in the extent to which they returned to pre-stroke levels of social activities. Socially isolated patients were an average of only 1 point down on their pre-stroke score, compared with a fall of 2.3 points among patients who reported no social isolation, but the difference was not statistically significant. It could be tentatively suggested that patients with a lower level

Table 33. *Views of patients and their supporters on changes since before the stroke*

Change	Patient getting about		Patient looking after self	
	Patients (%)	Supporters (%)	Patients (%)	Supporters (%)
Much less	58	61	26	35
Slightly less	25	15	35	21
No change/more	17	24	39	44
No. of respondents (= 100%)	76	75	77	75

of social functioning view themselves, in Hyman's (1972) terms, as having 'lesser need for successful rehabilitation because of social isolation ... [they] may see little point in strenuously exerting themselves in a rehabilitation program in order to produce greater achievement' (p. 95). This concern with returning to life as it was before the stroke, rather than in functional improvement for its own sake, reflects an orientation among patients and supporters towards 'return to normal'.

The views of patients and supporters about the extent to which patients had returned to 'normal' physical activities is shown in Table 33.

The views of patients and supporters on changes in the patient's mobility agreed in 63% of cases. Their assessments were clearly related to changes in the disability score. The proportion of patients who described themselves as getting about much less increased from 51% among patients who had returned to or improved upon their mobility score before the stroke, to 81% of patients whose score fell by 3 or more points. The supporters of patients whose mobility score had declined described 78% of them as getting about much less; but for patients who had returned to normal or even improved, 50% were still described by their supporters as getting about much less. Similarly only 23% of these (back to normal) patients described themselves as getting about on their own as much as before the stroke. Both patients and supporters thus view the decline in mobility as more extensive than shown by the measured change scores. There are possible reasons for this. To take walking as an example, the maximum score is for walking 50 yards independently; many patients may be walking less than they used to but still more than 50 yards. (Thirty per cent of this group of patients who previously walked outdoors 440 yards or more were, at 18 months, walking more than 50 yards independently but less than 440 yards outdoors.) The Barthel score may be used as a sensitive measure of change in dependence (Granger *et al.*, 1979), but it is not an adequate indicator of change in higher levels of performance.

There was no difference associated with the patient's age in the proportion who felt they were getting about less; but only 19% of people aged 80 or over said they were getting about much less, compared with 68% of younger patients. Similarly, it appears that middle-class patients may take a more serious view of change in mobility. All middle-class patients said they were getting about less, even those who had returned to or improved on their pre-stroke mobility score, but 22% of patients classified as working-class said there had been no change in getting about or they were doing more, and this proportion was 31% among patients who had returned to or improved on their mobility score before the stroke.

Patients and supporters were asked how much they felt the patient had changed in looking after himself or herself with regard to activities such as washing, dressing, feeding and using the toilet. The responses are shown in Table 33, and the two views agreed in 64% of cases. The views of both patients and supporters were closely related to measured change in self-care scores. The proportion of patients who felt they were doing as much as before the stroke fell from 76% of those who were recorded as having maintained or improved their performance down to none of those whose score on the self-care measure had fallen by 3 or more points. Eighty per cent of the supporters of patients who were doing the same or more than before the stroke said there had been no change, compared with 18% of the supporters of patients who were doing less. The good correlation between 'objective' and 'subjective' assessments of change probably reflects the nature of the activities such as washing and dressing, which tend to be done either independently or not, with no opportunity for extra performance above the rating for independence – though, of course, the patient could do something more or less easily or quickly.

Nor surprisingly the proportion of patients reporting that they were doing much less to care for themselves increased, from none of those who were rated as having no disability at 1 month after the stroke to 58% of those who were rated as having severe disability. There were no differences associated with the patient's age, marital status or social class, but men were more likely to view themselves as doing much less self-care; 47% of them said this compared with 13% of women. Among patients who were within one or two points of the self-care score they had before the stroke, 24% of men, compared with only 3% of women, felt they were looking after themselves much less.

There is no obvious reason why men should tend to overstate their loss of abilities in self-care, nor why younger patients and middle-class patients should feel they have deteriorated more in getting about since the stroke. Perhaps their perceptions refer to aspects of self-care or mobility that were not assessed, or it may be that the expectations of these groups are higher in some respects; it is not because they have dropped more points on the measured changes – the proportion of patients whose mobility deteriorated actually increased with age. The possibility that loss of independence is viewed as more problematic by these groups is taken up in the following sections after a description of longer-term physical disability.

Physical disability at 18 months after the stroke

In the longer term, at a mean of 18 months after the stroke, almost two-thirds of the patients were classified on their Barthel scores as having mild or no disability (see Table 26). However, as Table 28 showed, there remain high levels of dependency in some daily activities: less than half of the patients walked outside for 50 yards or more, or climbed a modest flight of stairs, or washed their body without help. Only one-fifth of patients travelled outside by car, bus or train on their own, and although two-thirds went as passengers in a car, 72% had not been on a bus or train in the 3 months before the third interview – a far greater restriction in use than found among the general population of older people (OPCS, 1982).

Mobility

Eighteen months after the stroke the average mobility score was 5.7 (out of a maximum of 8). It did not vary with the social class, marital status or sex of the patient, but patients aged 80 and over were less mobile, with an average score of 4.4 compared with 6.1 for patients aged 60–79. This difference is illustrated in the proportion of patients who walked outside 50 yards or more independently; this was 44% of people aged 60–79 but only 17% of people aged 80 and over. Altogether 13% of patients were unable to walk at all, but this did not vary with age. (Only 3 patients were unable to walk and unable to use a wheelchair, and 2 of these were in hospital with recent recurrent strokes.)

Age was not a factor influencing patients' views about their mobility. Altogether 26% of patients reported that they had a problem getting from room to room and 55% of patients said they had difficulty getting up and down stairs, but neither of these proportions was associated with the age or sex of the patients. As a summary of their views on current mobility, 26% of patients reported that getting about now caused them no problem, 35% that it was some problem and 39% that it was a great problem.

In general, the patients' views were related only to a rather gross division of the mobility scores: 63% of those with a score of 3 or less said getting about was a great problem, compared with 32% of patients who had a higher mobility score. Some of the reasons why patients described mobility as a problem appear straightforward: they may, for example, have been inclined to fall, or have been effectively housebound or wheelchair-bound and unable to get out. Some patients described the problem in terms of restrictions on their leisure activities. Two men, living in comfortable homes with their wives but generally able to get about only in a wheelchair, expressed their frustrations. One, whose main hobby was gardening, said:

Of course it is [a great problem]; it drives me round the bend. When I came home in the decent weather I thought 'I'll soon get over this.'

The other man reflected on his social life:

I don't consider that I get about much. I've not been further than 50 yards along the street. Never to the local [pub] for a beer or out with friends at all. I reckon I'm very restricted now.

The significance of getting about in order to pursue hobbies or interests was illustrated, too, by another middle-class man whose mobility score was 5 and who described getting about as 'some problem'.

But a lot of it is in the mind; when I think something is going to happen I anticipate it's going to happen and I'm all at sea. There's a certain problem – frustration. When I hear my neighbour knocking a nail in or sawing a piece of wood I think to myself 'You lucky fellow'. I used to do it all for myself. This sums it up [showed interviewer a cup with 'I'm a mug from Peckham' written on it] ... When I came home from hospital I'd thought I'd sling it out but I haven't done so, as you see.

The patients who viewed mobility as a problem often did so in relation to what they had done before or what others did. Two women, for example, both of whom scored the maximum (8) for mobility, described it as a 'slight problem':

See when I go out on my own, only to the shops, I can walk the speed I want to, but with anybody else they seem to be in a hurry.

I find it not [a problem] in the home, but if I go out I realise I can't carry heavy bags and if I'm not careful I might stumble. I notice I can't walk so far; you soon get tired.

Another two women, both of whom scored 8 on mobility, described getting about as a great problem because they expected to be able to do more, as had been their custom:

To me it's a big problem. I'm used to walking and getting about a lot. I've been home all this time and I'm not walking properly yet.

I can get about and hoover this house, but there are certain things I can't do, and these irritate me so much. Great problem to get out.

At the other extreme of dissonance between performance and perception are the patients who have little mobility but who do not view getting about as a problem. They tended to refer to themselves as not being the 'worrying type' or described worry as unproductive. For example, one woman who could get out of bed without help but needed her husband's support for everything else said mobility was no problem:

I don't think of it. I'm not a worrying person.

Similarly another woman, living in sheltered housing, who could walk less than 50 yards on her own said:

What's the good of worrying. You know you can't so you just get used to it. I sometimes walk in here [her living room] for exercise.

Perhaps this acceptance of limited mobility brought with it relief from worry about other responsibilities, or reflected, in part, resignation to some decline with old age. However, the proportion of patients who viewed mobility as a problem did not vary with age, marital status or sex of the patient. Social class was a factor, only 6% of middle-class patients feeling that getting about was no problem compared with 31% of working-class patients. Perhaps middle-class patients, more used to having some control over their destinies and to planning for the future, found it less easy to be fatalistic about the extent of their disability. The measured changes do not show that middle-class patients were either more disabled or made less recovery. But, as will be discussed in Chapter 8, middle-class patients were less likely to feel they had made a significant recovery and it may be that this group of patients felt the loss of mobility more keenly because they had more options and opportunities when they were mobile.

Self-care

At the third interview around 18 months after the stroke the average self-care score was 5.8 (out of a maximum of 8). This was not associated with the patient's sex, social class or age. In general, the proportion of patients who described looking after themselves as some problem or a great problem was clearly related to their self-care score; thus, for example, the proportion of patients who said it was a great problem to look after themselves fell from 40% of those with a self-care score of less than 4 to only 2% of patients whose score was 7 or 8. Altogether 54% of patients said looking after themselves was no problem, 25% described it as some problem and 21% as a great problem.

Several patients mentioned that they were 'glad to be able to do it' or that they would 'sooner do it' themselves. Being able to feed and wash and use the toilet independently has a symbolic importance which is probably greater than that for mobility; it is close to feelings of pride and dignity. As one woman who lived with her brother said:

It's an effort but I do it. I like looking after myself, keeping myself clean; I'm fussy.

So were most patients, although several mentioned that looking after themselves caused tiredness or breathlessness. A married woman was able to do everything for herself, although bathing had been:

... a bit of a struggle. When my leg had been bad [husband] has had to lift me out of the bath. I don't like to keep calling him, I'm not a pretty sight. He said when we got married I was like a mermaid, now I'm like a whale!

In general, she found looking after herself 'some problem':

It's the breathlessness that's the problem ... I wouldn't like to let myself go too much.

Her comments also illustrate how, even among married patients, there was a reluctance to become dependent on the supporter for some personal tasks such as bathing and using the toilet, and married patients were no more or less likely to have help with these tasks. Probably help with dressing is invested with less personal meaning of dependency, and it was evident that married patients were less likely to dress themselves independently: only 40% were doing this compared with 66% of other patients. This may simply be a product of having someone available to help with a job that is frustrating, tiring and a struggle to perform. However, married patients were less likely to be viewed by their supporters as reluctant to ask for help: only 37% of married patients were described like this compared with 64% of other patients. The very high proportion of married patients who were living at home with their supporter (spouse) probably contributed to this. It is perhaps surprising that a majority of all supporters (53%) described the patient as in some way reluctant to ask for help when needed; they referred to characteristics of the patient such as 'proud', 'stubborn', 'independent' and 'doesn't like bothering people'.

In some ways it appeared that losing independence in self-care was more threatening to patients than living with some loss of mobility. Patients would plan the night before and lay out clothes for the morning; they would use aids and develop ingenious ways of getting in and out of clothes or a bath; they were prepared to be slow, to start the same process many times, and to take extra precautions. When, after every effort, the patient remained dependent it was distressing. One woman was able only to use a receptacle herself in place of the toilet ('I've got a bucket and my daughter-in-law empties it at night'); not surprisingly, she viewed self-care as 'a great problem':

I try hard. No one knows how I try but it's hopeless. When I was in hospital they made me do it the best way I could. They said 'You are getting on fine', but you've got to in hospital. Nurses just come round and say 'How are you doing?' I'm fed up here being miserable. You want to have somewhere where you can talk to somebody. I've been up since 6.45 a.m. and I've got nothing in life. I wouldn't mind if I could do anything.

In the same way as for mobility, and probably for similar reasons, middle-class patients were more likely to describe looking after themselves as a problem: 69% of them said this compared with 39% of working-class patients. Neither married patients nor older patients were more or less likely to view looking after themselves as a problem, but 37% of men described it as a great problem compared with only 11% of women. This possibly explains why more men felt they were doing much less self-care. Men appeared to find dependency less easy to bear, perhaps because more of them lived together with other people who routinely witnessed the men's inability to care for themselves.

The patient's level of disability at 1 month after the stroke did not distinguish which patients would view getting about as a problem. But Barthel scores at 1 month were related to viewing self-care as a problem at 18 months after the stroke. The proportion of patients who described self-care as a problem increased from 17% of those who were classified as normal at 1 month up to 71% of patients who had a severe disability.

The health of patients and supporters

When patients were asked in their second and third interviews about their main health problem since the stroke, only a minority mentioned the stroke directly. In part, this was because the concept of health was not necessarily bound up with physical disability. A man who had endured a subsequent stroke and who was unable to walk said:

My health's alright; it's just that I can't walk about. I never have suffered with my health. I've always been a healthy chap.

Other patients, too, appeared to understand the question as taking the stroke for granted:

Just the stroke, nothing in my life before.

Many patients mentioned difficulties probably caused by the stroke but without referring back to that event. It was not easy to disentangle the effects of the stroke from many other health problems. For example, a man in his sixties who had been running his own business was aware of:

Oedema in my legs. Ulcers on my ankles for a very long time. My throat is sort of gone. I feel as if ... how can I explain it ... if I could talk better I'd explain it ... the point is I talk to people and I think I'm talking loud, but they just walk past; there's no noise coming out. I can't explain that. Of course, old Dr Bailey thinks I made a rapid recovery, marvellous, but I think they pushed me too hard.

And a woman in her eighties who lived with her son reported the common difficulty with getting about:

Walking; I don't know what's the matter with this blinkin' foot. I lose my balance a bit. I have to use the stick but that's no bother.

Patients with relatively slight physical disability appeared to focus more on their social and personal problems. Thus, for example, three women, all aged within a few years of 70, who had few health problems before the stroke and who were living at home were most concerned, 9 months after the stroke, by more general problems of getting through the day:

In the beginning I was very depressed, cried for nothing. But the doctor said you don't cry for nothing. It was something to do with my brain after the stroke. The doctor explained something to do with the fluids in the brain that weren't working to counteract each other. When I came home I couldn't sleep – right morbid. So he gave me anti-depression pills, not to stop me sleeping, but just in case I wake up in the night. It blocks the brain so if you wake up you don't start thinking.

Not boredom. I try not to get down in the dumps. I can't do things I want to do. I sit and knit. Doctor said yesterday I've got to take it easy. I'm bothered by my leg and hand from the stroke. And when the weather's cold and damp it seems to affect you more. See, often I can't feel anything in this hand.

I don't know what's wrong. I get up and I don't want to do anything. I feel just like a load of jelly. I can't get going. Suppose that's at my age, but when you've been active all your life, it comes a bit bad.

Table 34. *Patients'[a] assessments of health for their age before and after the stroke*

	Before stroke[b] (%)	9 months after stroke (%)	18 months after stroke (%)
Excellent	33	3	9
Good	38	44	44
Fair	25	36	28
Poor	4	17	19
No. of patients (= 100%)	84	84	79

[a] Survivors to 18 months after the stroke.
[b] Reported 1 month after the stroke.

Most patients when talking about their general health referred to a variety of problems common among older people: eyes, feet, breathlessness, lack of energy, angina, arthritis, ulcers, controlling water, and digestion were mentioned. In terms of their general health the stroke may not always have been the main problem but, half of the survivors at 18 months after the stroke rated their health less positively than they had rated their general health before the stroke. (This was investigated in the first interview and reported in Chapter 2.) Table 34 shows that only 9% of the longer-term survivors assessed their health as excellent, whereas 33% of them had done so in relation to life before the stroke.

Patients at all levels of self-assessment referred to a variety of health problems, some of which were long-standing while others were associated with the stroke. The existence of disability did not obviate a positive assessment of general health; for example, a woman aged 79 who spent most of her time in a wheelchair described herself as in 'excellent health':

... but I seem to have got to the stage now where I don't feel I'm getting any better. I can walk, do things without these contraptions, but I don't seem to improve. I've given up on this hand; it doesn't seem to be any better, but you don't know.

However, for many patients the stroke, subsequent disability and changes in their life were all seen in relation to their previous performance and current age. A woman in her sixties said:

Well, I mean it won't be as good as it was before, and on the other hand you're getting older.

Many others also describe their health as good, considering their age:

Not improving a lot. I'm just looking for the warmer weather. For 78 years of age, good. Up to that Sunday when I had this stroke I was doing all my own gardening, now I do none of it.

I just wish I could walk and get out a bit. That's the main problem. Not bad at all for my age [80]. They say to me you don't look your age, but I say sometimes I feel it.

Age was not a factor that related to the patients' general assessments of their health, unlike at the first interview when patients aged 60–79 had taken a more negative view of their health before the stroke. The greater propensity of women for describing their health as only fair or poor persisted, albeit that the difference was not quite statistically significant and applied only among those patients aged 60–79: 56% of the women described their health as fair or poor compared with 32% of the men. The patients who described their health for their age as poor were particularly inclined to view themselves as having a great problem getting about: 93% of them felt this, but only 25% of other patients. The general relationship between the rating of disability, in terms of the Barthel score, and the patient's assessment of his or her health was consistent, such that the proportion of patients with mild or no disability fell from 100% of those rating themselves as in excellent health to 53% of those who described their health 18 months after the stroke as poor.

Among supporters, there was no change between the first and third interviews in the proportion who rated their health for their age as excellent, good, fair or poor. The main difference at 18 months was that sex differences were found in all age groups, so that altogether 58% of women but only 17% of male supporters rated their health for their age as fair or poor. Rating of health was not associated with the supporter's age, nor was it related either to the severity of the patient's disability or to living with the patient.

Results from analysis of the aspects of health investigated in the Nottingham Health Profile reinforced the findings in the general statements that the health of women supporters 18 months after the stroke was worse than that of the men. There was no consistent relationship between scores on the profile and the age or social class of the supporter, nor were these scores related to the severity of the patient's disability. In all respects, though, as Table 35 shows, a higher proportion of women supporters identified problems. This association between health and the sex of the supporter was not restricted to supporters with a specific relationship to the patient, but was a general finding.

Table 35. *Sex of the supporter related to the reporting of health problems.*

	Proportion with any problem	
Aspect of health	Men (%)	Women (%)
Energy	18	48
Pain	0	40
Emotion	23	62
Sleep	9	58
Social isolation	5	26
Physical mobility	0	46
No. of supporters (= 100%)	22	50

When the change in health scores is considered, the general picture is one with very little direction, such that on all the dimensions except 'emotional distress' most supporters have the same score (nought) that they had a month after the stroke. Table 36 presents the results for all supporters. However, the pattern of changes was quite different for men and women, such that female supporters were more likely than men to be bothered to an increased extent by problems with all aspects of health, and significantly so with: pain (scores for 33% of women had increased but for none of the men); emotional distress (38% of women compared with 13% of men); sleep (31% compared with 4%); and physical mobility (27% compared with 0). These increasing problems were experienced in fairly equal measure by both women who did and who did not live with the stroke patient. Only with regard to sleep did the health of women living with the patient deteriorate more than that of others: 52% of women living with the patient experienced an increase in sleeping problems, compared with 12% of women supporters who did not live with the patient.

Unfortunately, these changes in health could be monitored only after the stroke, so that comparisons reflect change between 1 and 18 months after the event. However, when, at the third interview, supporters were asked whether they felt their health had been affected by the stroke 38% thought it had, and described the consequences mainly in terms of worry, exhaustion and mental strain. This proportion was not related to the severity of the patient's disability, to whether the supporter lived with the patient or to the supporter's age or social class. However, only 13% of the men felt their health had been affected compared with 49% of women,

Table 36. *Changes in the supporters' scores on the Nottingham Health Profile from 1 to 18 months after the stroke*

Change in score	Aspect of health					
	Energy (%)	Pain (%)	Emotion (%)	Sleep (%)	Isolation (%)	Mobility (%)
+3 or more	0	4	8	4	0	3
+1 or 2	24	19	21	18	13	15
No change	66	72	48	58	83	67
−1 or 2	10	4	20	20	4	15
−3 or less	0	1	3	0	0	0
No. of supporters (=100%)	70	71	71	71	71	71

reflecting a general difference in the experience of caring for a patient with a stroke that is discussed in detail in the following chapters.

SUMMARY

Survival   Deaths among the patients continued at a high level for the period between 1 and 3 months after the stroke: 22% of the patients died, including more than half of those who had been very severely disabled. Altogether 36% of the patients died between 1 and 12 months after the stroke. The patient's poorer mental state, assessed as both cognitive impairment and emotional distress, was strongly associated with mortality. As in other studies, older patients were more likely to die, but this pattern was not statistically significant after controlling for severity of the disability.

Physical recovery   Disability as an outcome should be distinguished from functional improvement and return to normal, because, for example, the patients who make the most functional improvement following the stroke are also the most disabled. Most improvement takes place in the first few months after the stroke, and, in terms of Barthel scores, is complete by 6 or 9 months after the stroke. Between 9 and 18 months after the stroke there was a small decline in disability scores, particularly for self-care activities and particularly among patients aged 80 or over. Severity of disability at 1 month after the stroke was clearly related to subsequent improvement. Among patients with moderate or severe disability, the patient's mood – feelings of social isolation and emotional distress – was related to functional improvement, with less distressed and more socially engaged patients doing better. In other respects, for example marital status and household size, there were no differences in functional improvement following the stroke. It is suggested that patients with a lower level of social activity before the stroke may view themselves as having less need for successful rehabilitation.

Altogether, by 18 months after the stroke only 1 patient in 3 had returned to the same level of (lack of) physical disability that existed before the stroke; this was less likely among older patients and those who had been more disabled by the stroke. The views of patients and supporters about the extent to which patients had returned to normal tended to parallel 'objective' assessments, but older patients were likely to perceive less change in mobility, while men tended to see more deterioration in their self-care abilities.

By 18 months after stroke two-thirds of patients were classified as having mild or no disability; but Barthel scores tend to camouflage high levels of dependency in some daily activities: three-quarters of the patients were dependent in some activity incorporated in the disability rating. More patients felt they had problems with getting about than with looking after themselves and several expressed particular relief that they were able to wash themselves and use the toilet without help. Middle-class patients were more likely to view their dependence as a problem. It may be that patients who had been used to having control over their activities and who had had more opportunities available to them found it less easy to accept dependence and restricted choices in everyday life.

Health of patients and supporters   A majority of patients discussed their health in relation to common disorders of the elderly and without referring directly to the stroke. Those with little physical disability focused more on their social and personal problems. However, half the patients rated their health 18 months after the stroke less positively than they had done for their general health before the stroke. Their assessments were clearly related to disability scores, but their age and sex were much less important factors than they had been in ratings of health before the stroke. Among the supporters, however, women rated their health at 18 months after the stroke more negatively than did men, and this sex difference was reflected generally in reports of health problems recorded in the Nottingham Health Profile. The health of women supporters, whether they did or did not live with the patient, appeared to have deteriorated much more than that of the men. Altogether, half the female supporters but only 1 in 8 of the men felt their health had been affected by the stroke, primarily through worry, exhaustion or mental strain.

CHAPTER SIX

Support in the community

Following the stroke, most patients in Greenwich were admitted to hospital and stayed there for several weeks; only 10% of the patients who survived to 9 months after the stroke were still in hospital then. The length of time for which patients were in hospital was clearly associated with the severity of their disability at 1 month after the stroke; this is shown in Table 37.

None of the patients who had lived at home with a spouse remained in hospital throughout the first 9 months (although some were subsequently re-admitted); this may be compared with 14% of patients in all other households, and 53% of those without a spouse who were severely or very severely disabled. Patients who lived alone were not generally more likely to stay in hospital longer than other patients, but patients aged 80 or over were more likely to be in hospital for the first 9 months – 23% compared with 4% of younger patients. This age difference fell below significance if only patients without spouses were considered (23% of patients aged 80 or over compared with 8% of those aged 60–79 were in hospital for all of the first 9 months after the stroke).

There were no differences in duration of stay in the hospital associated with the patient's sex or social class, or with the type of accommodation (private, council) that the patients had lived in before the stroke.

Leaving hospital

From the viewpoint of patients, there were few who had problems over their discharge from hospital. Among survivors at the second interview only 9 patients (12%) said there was a lack of time for some necessary arrangements to be made – principally provision of aids or services. A 72-year old man with mild disability was discharged to his own house, but was unhappy about:

Table 37. *Duration of hospital stay related to patients' severity of disability*

Length of hospital stay	Barthel rating				
	Severe (9 or less) (%)	Moderate (10–14) (%)	Mild (15–19) (%)	Normal (20) (%)	All hospital patients (%)
Less than 4 weeks	11	38	52	92	40
4 but less than 8 weeks	11	31	31	0	19
8 but less than 12 weeks	9	6	10	8	9
12 weeks or more	43	25	7	0	22
All time since stroke	26	0	0	0	10
No. of patients (= 100%)	35	16	29	13	93

The aids – like the stair bannister took 6 weeks. I went up and down the stairs on my hands and knees for 4 weeks, and by the time the bannister came it was almost too late – I was back to normal again.

Just a few patients complained that the home help or the Meals on Wheels (home meals) service failed to arrive on the day they went home, but these problems appeared to be resolved within a day or two. Of course the supporters were often involved in sorting out difficulties and it was apparent in some of these interviews that the patient's satisfaction did not represent the supporter's feelings about discharge – but supporters were not asked directly about this.

A small proportion (5%) of patients reported that they were unhappy to have stayed in hospital for the time they did and wished they had been discharged sooner. A further 7% of patients said they wished they could have stayed longer in hospital, mainly because they felt they were not well enough to come home or because they felt they could have benefited from more therapy.

A few patients remarked that they were more comfortable in hospital than at home; and among the large majority (88%) who were happy to leave hospital when they did, several commented that the food, comforts or company were better in hospital. A woman who returned to living alone in a three-bedroomed house remarked:

I was glad to get home – sorry to leave the company behind. I mean some were quite nice. And it was nice to talk to the nurses. You miss that.

Home

All the patients who were to return to living at home had done so before the second interview, 9 months after the stroke. At 1 month after the stroke only 30% of patients were interviewed in their own home, but this proportion was 87% at the second interview. Subsequently some patients were re-admitted to hospital, while others established themselves in residential care or a nursing home. Altogether 86% of patients were interviewed in their own home, in the community, at 18 months after the stroke. These proportions are very much the same as reported in previous studies (Brocklehurst *et al.*, 1978a; Weddell and Beresford, 1979). However, the place of interview and the patient's definition of the place where he or she lived are different for a small number of patients: some of those seen in hospital 18 months after the stroke were in permanent care, but others maintained a home in the community or said they were waiting for a place in residential care; several patients had been re-admitted for specific problems, and one was a woman who had suffered a serious stroke only days before the interview.

Only 6% of patients were classified as permanently in a hospital or nursing home, and 8% as living in a residential home for the elderly. The 'permanent' homes of patients who were seen 18 months after the stroke and their category of accommodation before the stroke are shown in Table 38.

A quarter (24%) of the patients were living in a different category of accommodation 18 months after the stroke, mainly because 9 patients (10%) had moved into sheltered housing and 9 (10%) had gone into institutional care (hospital, nursing home or residential home for the elderly). The factors influencing return home and type of accommodation are many and they interact with each other (Feigenson *et al.*, 1977a). Previous studies have suggested that older patients (Isaacs and Marks, 1973), those with more severe disability (Granger *et al.*, 1979), with poorer mental functioning (Isaacs and Marks, 1973; Feigenson *et al.*, 1977a) and with inadequate family support (Lehmann *et al.*, 1975a) are more likely to remain in institutional care. The number of longer-term survivors in this study who remained in hospital or institutional care was small (12). Among those who had previously lived in the community (of whom 9 patients were subsequently in institutional care), neither age, severity of disability at 1 month after the stroke nor Walkey (orientation) score was related, at a statistically significant level, to moving into institutional care. However, 20% of the patients who had been living alone in the community before their stroke went into institutional care compared with only

Table 38. *Type of accommodation patients had before the stroke and 18 months later*

Accommodation	Before stroke (%)	18 months after the stroke (%)
Owner-occupied	29	28
Council	36	29
Privately rented	8	4
Sheltered housing	13	21
Lives with family or friends	10	4
Residential home	3	8
Hospital or nursing home	1	6
No. of patients (= 100%)	92	92

3% of the patients who had been living with their spouse. And while the patient's initial level of disability appeared unimportant, the level of persisting disability 18 months after the stroke was a factor, so that the proportion who had moved into institutional care fell from a third of those with severe disability to none of those without disability.

The importance of local authority housing is emphasised in Greenwich by the movement of patients into sheltered housing. This was home at 18 months after the stroke for 17% of married patients as well as 29% of widowed patients. Following the stroke, none of the patients who owned their own houses moved into sheltered housing compared with 16% of the patients who had been in council or privately rented accommodation, or who had lived in the home of family or friends. At 18 months after the stroke 27% of patients classified as working-class were living in sheltered housing, but none of those classified as middle-class.

These comparisons of housing before and after the stroke do not capture the full extent of the actual changes in accommodation, since some patients moved within the categories while others moved but died during the 18 months after the stroke. Table 39 summarises change and preferences for change between the three stages of the study.

Only one patient moved twice – first into the home of her son and his family, and then with them to a house outside London which had a separate accommodation for the patient. Forty-one per cent of patients who said at the second interview 9 months after the stroke that they had thought of moving had done so by the third interview at 18 months, compared with only 8% of the patients who said they had not thought of moving. There was some indication that owner-occupiers were less able or

Table 39. *Patients who had moved accommodation or thought of doing so*

	From before stroke to 9 months after stroke (%)	From 9 to 18 months after stroke (%)
Moved	13	16
Stayed but had thought of moving	21	20
Stayed and had not thought of moving	58	54
Stayed and don't know thoughts	8	10
No. of patients (= 100%)	108	93

willing to move than patients who were in rented accommodation: only 4% of people who owned their own homes moved before the second interview compared with 19% of people in council or privately rented accommodation. The difference is not quite statistically significant, nor were owner-occupiers more likely to say they had thought of moving. Possibly, then, owner-occupiers were simply more satisfied with their housing or more attached to where they lived as part of their self-identity. The adequacy of the different categories of accommodation is considered below.

Suitability of the housing

Among patients who moved house between the second and the third interviews 58% described their new accommodation with a higher rating of suitability than their previous abode. Satisfaction with moving no doubt reflects the reasons for the move and the new destination.

Patients and supporters had rather different views about the benefits of moving and about the suitability of the patient's housing. These views are shown in Table 40.

Just over half (53%) of the patients and supporters agreed in their ratings of the suitability of housing, and this proportion was the same among patients and supporters who lived together. Owner-occupied and council housing were rated more highly by patients than supporters, but there was no significant difference in the rating of these main housing types among either patients or supporters. Furthermore, both patients and supporters tended to give institutional care a poor rating for suitability. The housing of patients with moderate or severe disability was

Table 40. *The suitability of housing for patients: the views of patients and supporters*

Housing is:	Patients' views				Supporters' views			
	C/O[a] (%)	SH (%)	H/N/R (%)	All (%)	C/O (%)	SH (%)	H/N/R (%)	All (%)
Very suitable	61	82	25	61	38	100	44	49
Fairly suitable	31	18	50	30	47	0	12	35
Rather unsuitable	8	0	25	9	15	0	44	16
No. of patients (= 100%)	48	17	8	80	45	14	9	75

[a] C/O, council or owner-occupied housing; SH, sheltered housing; H/N/R, hospital, nursing home, residential home for the elderly.

generally more likely to be regarded as 'rather unsuitable': 20% of these patients said this compared with only 4% of less disabled patients; and 32% of the supporters of patients with moderate or severe disability thought the patient's housing was rather unsuitable compared with only 7% of the supporters of patients who had mild or no disability. The supporters of these disabled patients were particularly unhappy about accommodation for patients in a hospital or nursing home, 80% of which was described as rather unsuitable compared with 18% of the housing of other patients who had moderate or severe disability.

The responses of patients and supporters to a general question about their views on the patient's housing arrangements emphasised again the significance of the patient being able to get about in the house. Supporters, in particular, talked about problems with stairs and steps. The stairs were a barrier to going outside the home for some patients, while for others they were a barrier that clearly divided the house. The wives of two patients described the move to a downstairs bedroom for their husbands:

He sleeps downstairs now. About October I nearly fell downstairs bringing him down, so we don't bother anymore.

Oh, everything's alright. He sleeps downstairs as he can't get upstairs.

A patient who now slept downstairs remarked that his housing was:

Bloody awful, but I don't want to go away anywhere else.

Altogether, 54% of patients and 50% of the supporters reported that the patient had some difficulty at home managing steps or stairs. Among both groups, the housing of patients who had problems with the stairs was significantly more likely to be described as rather unsuitable than was the housing of patients who had no problems – 17% of the patients who reported problems with stairs said their housing was rather unsuitable but none of the other patients said this; the corresponding proportions for supporters were 30% and none.

Among patients with problems getting about the house, some move, others accommodate and many have aids or adaptations fitted to improve performance or safety. Half of the patients reported some adaptation made to their home or some aids (from bannisters and bath rails to cutlery and carpet holders) installed. Similar to the comments over discharge from hospital, only 9% of patients complained that there was any delay or difficulty over these aids or adaptations. Patients who were moderately or severely disabled a month after the stroke were more likely to have adaptations to their home or aids (74% compared with 28% of less disabled patients). There were no differences between stroke unit patients and those who had been on other wards over the provision or perceived usefulness of aids (cf. M. Smith *et al.*, 1981). A large majority of patients, even 18 months after the stroke, found their aids or adaptations useful; only 18% said that any of these aids were not useful. However, no simple relationship between provision of aids or adaptations and suitability of the patient's home was either expected or found.

Among the other main factors which appeared to influence the judgements on the suitability of the patient's housing was heating. Altogether 27% of supporters but only 12% of patients reported that the patient had difficulty in meeting the costs of heating. However, 26% of patients living in property rented either from the council or privately said they had problems paying for the heating, compared with only 6% of other patients.

Twenty-four hour supervision was another concern, and for the supporters it was a further attraction of sheltered housing. The anxieties about stroke and the need for help in an emergency had encouraged patients and families to install telephones. It is not known how many households had a telephone before the stroke, but 18 months later 70% had one, and the figure was 90% if patients in institutional care and sheltered housing are excluded (compared with 61% of households containing an elderly person reported from the Office of Population Censuses and Surveys, 1982). Only one patient said she had no system for summoning help in an emergency.

Supporters also noted that travelling to see the patient every day was a problem, not only for them but for patients who were dependent on their help. A woman who lived outside Greenwich but who cared for her housebound uncle said:

I wish he'd go in a place with a warden. When I can't get there and the home help doesn't go he's stuck there without food.

A supporter who lived in Kent commented on his mother's housing situation:

It's no good. There's one room that she can manage to get about in. There's no toilet facilities, no water. She can't have a proper wash unless the home help brings a bowl of water for her.

This woman lived in the front room of the family house with bed, commode, chair and television within three paces of each other. She lived alone, as did half the patients who, 18 months after the stroke, were living outside institutions. Among patients living in the community, the proportions living alone were 31% of those in owner-occupied housing, 52% of people in council accommodation and 74% of patients in sheltered housing.

In comparison with patients from other studies a higher proportion of patients in Greenwich were living alone. (For example, data on use of services will be compared with results from the Bristol study (Legh-Smith *et al.*, 1986) in which only 21% of patients in the community lived alone.) Household composition was largely a function of the patient's sex and age: 60% of women lived alone compared with 28% of men; and 61% of men were living with their spouse, compared with 18% of women. The proportion of patients living alone increased from 17% of patients aged 60–69 to 65% of those aged 80 or over; and the proportion living with their spouse fell from 54% of those in their sixties to 4% of patients aged 80 and over. Household composition was not associated with the patient's social class.

Sources of help and support

The structure of support at home and in the community is a critical element in maintaining, and in maintaining the quality of life of, patients in the community. Much has been written about the use and availability of different sorts of help for stroke patients (e.g. Weddell and Beresford, 1979; Garraway *et al.*, 1981*b*; Legh-Smith *et al.*, 1986), but the focus has been on statutory services and there is very little to indicate whether patients find the services useful or lacking in some way. Although several studies have considered the implications for carers of the current distribution of services (Jones and Vetter, 1985; Legh-Smith *et al.*, 1986), the focus has been on the consequences of services to patients – the

Table 41. *Sources of help for getting about among patients at home 9 months after the stroke, by sex of patient*

Source of help	Men (%)	Women (%)	All (%)
No one	41	34	37
Son/daughter	22	38	32
Spouse	38	14	23
Nurse	0	2	1
Other	24	33	29
No. of patients (= 100%)	37	58	95

Percentages add to more than 100% because some patients reported help from more than one source.

experiences of carers and their preferences for different services or sources of support have been relatively neglected.

The 'informal' sector of care – family, friends and neighbours – forms the backbone of support provided to patients. In particular, the availability of supporters living with the patient appears to have a profound effect on the use of formal services (e.g. Legh-Smith *et al.*, 1986). This chapter therefore considers the different sources of support available to patients and supporters – family and friends, community health and social services – and assesses from whom patients and supporters derived most assistance after the stroke.

Support for patients

Getting about

At the second interview, 9 months after the stroke, patients were asked who, during the previous month, had helped them with getting about indoors, up or down stairs, or outside. Among patients at home, a little over one-third reported that no one had helped them: this included 77% of the patients with no disability but none of those who were classified as severely disabled. Sons and daughters were mentioned by a third of the patients as helping them to get about and this proportion was similar for patients who lived alone and with others, but while none of the former group reported help from a spouse, 36% of patients who lived with others said this. One consequence of the sex difference in household composition (many more men living with their spouse) appears to be different patterns of family support for getting about. This is shown in Table 41, which also indicates a relatively modest contribution from health service staff; the 'other' category is composed mainly of friends and other relatives, but includes ambulancemen, care assistants and physiotherapists.

Altogether 81% of patients in the community felt they were receiving enough help to get about and 15% that they needed more help; 4% made some other comment. These proportions were not related to the sources of support, or to the severity of the patient's disability, age, sex or household composition.

Self-care

At this second interview patients living in the community were asked a similar question about who, during the last month, had helped them with feeding, dressing, bathing or using the toilet. There is less involvement of the patient's children in helping with self-care activities and much greater participation of health services staff, in particular district nurses and bathing assistants. The figures in Table 42 show this, as well as the high proportion of disabled patients who receive help from their spouse with looking after themselves.

Since most of the spouses are wives, it is not surprising that men and women differ in their main sources of support: 51% of men report receiving help with self-care from a spouse, but only 17% of women. Women patients were not more likely to be receiving help from sons or daughters, nor were there any differences by sex of the patient in the provision of support by district nurses and bathing assistants. Women were using more help from 'other' sources, including sisters, friends and the home help (particularly, it seemed, with dressing).

Twelve per cent of patients felt that they needed more help with self-care, a proportion that was not related to the patient's age, sex or severity of disability.

Psychosocial support

The need among patients for morale-boosting support, as well as practical help, was discussed in Chapter 4. In the interview at 9 months after the stroke all patients were asked questions concerning emotional distress and social isolation, and then asked who had been there for them since the

Table 42. *Severity of patients' disability related to sources of help with self-care at 9 months after the stroke*

	Barthel rating				
Source of help	Severe (5–9) (%)	Moderate (10–14) (%)	Mild (15–19) (%)	Normal (20) (%)	All patients
No one	0	10	24	88	36
Son/daughter	9	25	21	0	15
Spouse	73	55	26	0	31
Nurse	36	15	8	0	11
Bath assistant	9	25	24	4	17
Other	18	35	26	8	22
No. of patients (= 100%)	11	20	38	26	95

Percentages add to more than 100% because some patients reported help from more than one source.

Table 43. *Sources of psychosocial support, by sex of patient*

	Men (%)	Women (%)	All patients (%)
Sources of emotional support:			
No one	26	20	22
Spouse	59	10	27
Son/daughter	26	36	32
Other	33	44	40
No. of patients (= 100%)	27	50	77
Sources of social support:			
No one	17	22	20
Spouse	50	9	24
Son/daughter	27	51	42
Other	27	31	29
No. of patients (= 100%)	30	55	85

Percentages add to more than 100% because some patients reported support from more than one source.

stroke to provide emotional and social support.* The patient's responses, presented in Table 43, show that four-fifths of patients did have support, but that the sources differed considerably between men and women. Men identified their spouse as by far the most important source of both emotional and social support. The proportion of women who mentioned their children (which most had) as a source of emotional support was about the same as the proportion who referred to friends, sisters and grandchildren (the 'other' category). But children appear to make a more significant contribution to enhancing the social esteem of women patients.

The proportion of patients who felt that no one had given them emotional or social support was not related to the patient's age or severity of disability. There were no simple relationships between levels of emotional distress and reported support. This is not surprising since some patients who were not at all distressed explained they had had no reason to use support while other patients with high levels of support exclaimed that having no one they could talk to was part of the problem.

Who helped most?

Family support is the main source of help for patients, and the supporter is usually the closest relative available to the patient. At the third interview, 18 months after the stroke, patients offered a summary view on which single person they felt had done most to help them since the stroke. Only 7% of patients said that no one had, but 32% identified their spouse, 39% a child, 9% a friend, 6% a sibling and 6% mentioned someone else (including one rehabilitation therapist and two care attendants) and 1% did not know who had done most. Eighty-seven per cent of patients who lived with their spouse identified the spouse as the main helper; of the people who lived alone 58% identified a child as the main source of support, 13% said a friend or neighbour and 5% a sibling. (Among those living alone in the community, i.e. not in an institution, 71% said they received most help and support from children and 16% said from siblings.) As expected, 65% of men but only 12% of women identified a spouse as the person who had done most to help them – though where a spouse existed there was no difference between men and women in the proportion who identified the spouse as the main helper.

* The questions were: (a) Since your stroke illness, when sometimes you (may) have felt a bit upset or fed up, has anyone – from your family, friends, or anyone else – been around to cheer you up or raise your spirits? (b) Since your stroke illness, when sometimes you (may) have felt alone or a bit cut off from other people, has anyone – from your family, friends or anyone else – been around to show you how much you are valued and how important you are to them?

Adequacy of family support

Few patients believe, or at least express the feeling, that they should be receiving more help from their family or friends. Only 18% of patients, when asked 18 months after the stroke, said that they thought any family, friends or neighbours should have helped more: none mentioned their spouse, 3 patients each identified a son or daughter, neighbours, or a sister who could have done more, while 1 referred to the family in general.

Patients tended to feel that family members or friends who were mentioned could have shown more general interest rather than that they could have performed a lot of specific tasks. With their neighbours there seemed to be disappointment that they did not think to make small gestures which the patients felt would not have been an inconvenience. One housebound woman living alone felt that the neighbours:

... don't bother. It wouldn't hurt them to call in, ask if you needed anything. They don't trouble. [Interviewer: Why not?] They think the home help will do everything. I suppose if I asked her [neighbour] she would go shopping for me, but it wouldn't hurt to call in.

The failure of others to help for over a year or more following the stroke sometimes generated bitterness. An 80-year-old woman, with mild disability but living alone on a hilly street, recalled:

When I first came out I felt very resentful of people who had cars but never came to offer help. [Interviewer: Why do you think they didn't help more?] I think they thought I was going to be very dependent on them and they weren't prepared even though I used to be in their house as much as my own. I think as well when you look perfectly alright ... My sister, she's never done anything; she said her responsibility was to her husband, and not to me. I've never forgotten that.

Most people, though, did not expect more help from their neighbours or anyone else. Some of the patients' comments were enthusiastic about this informal support, but a large proportion reflected feelings that it was better to be independent (as a household, not only as a patient), that others do as much as they can considering they have their own problems, or that there was not really anyone else available to do more because, for example, the relatives were dead or lived far away.

The number of patients who felt they should have been receiving more help was small; only 5% of patients without disability wanted more help, compared with 28% of others. None of the differences between patients with different demographic characteristics was statistically significant. The clearest of these differences was between patients living alone, 26% of whom felt family or neighbours could have helped more, and patients living with others, 10% of whom felt this.

Support for supporters

Sources of practical help

The main sources of support for the supporters of stroke patients include a higher proportion of professionals from the health and social services than was the case for the patients themselves. This may be because supporters require more discrete rather than continuous support, and because their own main supporter before the stroke might have been the patient. At the interview 18 months after the stroke supporters were asked who, if anyone, had helped them most by giving practical help. Altogether 31% said that no one had helped them. However, as Table 44 shows, this proportion fell from 50% of the supporters of patients who were not dependent to only 9% of the supporters of patients who still had severe disability.

The proportion of supporters who mentioned health and social services as the major source of practical support fell steadily with greater independence of the patients, although the decline was not statistically significant. Altogether, 7% of supporters mentioned the home help, 4% a social worker and 3% each mentioned the district nurse, care attendant and a doctor as their main source of support. The relationship of the supporter to the patient was important insofar as the patients were not generally giving the supporter practical help! Forty-four per cent of patients' spouses identified one of their children as the main source of practical support compared with 3% of patients identifying one of their own children in this way. The main sources of practical help for sons or daughters of the patient were the community services (mentioned by 30%) and their spouse (mentioned by 27%); only 7% reported that a brother or sister had given them most help.

Need for family support

Male supporters appeared to feel less need for the help and support of family and friends. At least this is what they expressed when asked directly at 9 months after the stroke how much, over the previous month, they had felt they needed support from family and friends. The differences are shown in Table 45.

This sex difference is mainly because 88% of the sons of patients felt

Table 44. *Severity of patients' disability at 18 months after the stroke related to sources of most practical help to the supporters*

	Barthel rating				
Main source of help to supporters:	Severe (5–9) (%)	Moderate (10–14) (%)	Mild (15–19) (%)	Normal (20) (%)	All supporters (%)
No one	9	19	34	50	31
Spouse	18	6	14	25	15
Child	36	38	17	13	24
Friend/neighbour	0	13	21	6	13
Sibling	0	0	10	6	6
Services	45	31	28	13	28
No. of supporters (= 100%)	11	16	29	16	72

Percentages may add to more than 100% if the supporter mentioned more than one main source of help.

Table 45. *Expressed need for family support in the previous month, by sex of the supporter*

Family support needed:	Male (%)	Female (%)	All supporters (%)
A lot	13	27	22
Some	9	16	14
A little	3	13	9
None at all	75	44	55
No. of supporters (= 100%)	32	63	95

they had no need for support from family and none of them felt they needed a lot of support. This may be the result of the sons doing less, but the explanation appears more complex than that since the need for family support was not related to either living with the patient or the severity of the patient's disability. Men, especially younger men, are likely to be physically stronger than women supporters, and probably more were car drivers, which would reduce their feelings of need for support from others. And perhaps men have different attitudes to the use of family, as opposed to state, support – an issue which has begun to attract systematic investigation (Allen *et al.*, 1987).

Table 46. *Relationship of supporters to patients, related to supporters'*
views that family or friends could have helped more

| | Relationship to patient | | All supporters |
	Spouse	Child	
9 months after stroke	26% (34)[a]	49% (39)	36% (95)
18 months after stroke	4% (26)	50% (32)	28% (74)

[a] Figures in brackets are the numbers upon which percentages are based.

Adequacy of family support

Dissatisfactions among the children of patients, including sons and daughters equally, dominate expressions of inadequacy in family support. Their frustrations about lack of help with caring were, as Table 46 shows, greater than among patients' spouses and did not diminish with time. Perhaps spouses can accommodate more readily since the patient is probably the main responsibility in their lives and they define themselves as the natural focus for support; most of the patients' sons and daughters, on the other hand, were married with their own families, and also with siblings who may not have shouldered their share of the continuing responsibility for caring.

At 18 months after the stroke three-quarters of the supporters who wanted more family help were sons or daughters of patients, and most of them (69% of those who felt they should have been helped more) wanted more support from their brothers and sisters.

A son who called into his mother's home on the way to and from work thought his siblings had neglected both him and his mother:

The rest of the family – two brothers and sisters – they disappeared when she came out of hospital. I got her on the phone [had it installed], but they never phone her. She feels it that they don't phone. [Interviewer: Why do you think they didn't help more?] They've got their own lives to lead and that's it. I'm the nearest.

Sons and daughters of patients painted a picture of other siblings who were selfish and uncaring. Among the explanations given for their siblings' lack of support were:

[Brother] loses patience because he thinks she should have gone in a home and she wouldn't; so that's it as far as he's concerned. And he finds it hard to see her like that and thinks it's best to stay away.

[Siblings] live in a world of their own. They can't be bothered; don't want to know.

[Brother] is in Darlington. I feel hard done by. He was always her golden boy. She rejected me. Now he doesn't care where she is as long as it's not with him.

These instances appear to reflect a feeling among some of the sons and daughters of patients that they have had to shoulder all the responsibility for caring, while their indolent brothers and sisters are free. However, this sense of injustice did not refer to having to do all the practical caring, rather that the supporter felt the siblings could 'visit a bit', 'go and see [the patient] more often', 'pop up and see her', 'bother to phone' and 'go over there, take her some flowers'. Supporters who felt their family could be doing more to help wanted them to show more 'caring interest' for the patient. Neither patients nor supporters appeared to feel that there was a significant shortfall in practical help.

Health and social services: services for patients

Among patients living in the community there is marked continuity in the use of community services. Between 9 and 18 months after the stroke only 1 patient stopped receiving a home help, while 2 patients started; 3 people gave up Meals on Wheels and 4 patients started taking them; 3 patients were seeing the district nurse at 18 months after the stroke when they had not seen her at 9 months, and 4 patients were no longer seeing the district nurse. The proportion of patients receiving these services at 9 and 18 months after the stroke is shown in Table 47.

In comparison with stroke patients in the Bristol stroke study many more of those in Greenwich were receiving support from home helps and Meals on Wheels. This may reflect provision of services, but the authors of the Bristol study concluded that the services were being provided for the patients who needed them most. However, patients in the Greenwich sample are older and more of them live alone – characteristics both associated with greater use of these services.

Among patients living at home, those who lived on their own received the majority of the services: three-quarters or more of those having home helps and Meals on Wheels lived alone. Among patients living alone, 78% received the home help service and 47% had Meals on Wheels, compared with 22% and 7% for the respective services among patients who lived with others. Only one man was using Meals on Wheels compared with 38% of women at home, and while 60% of women were receiving the home help service only 26% of men were. The proportion of patients having Meals on Wheels increased with age, from 5% of patients in their sixties to 46% of those aged 80 or over, and while 19% of patients aged 60–69 were receiving support from the home help this proportion was

Table 47. *Use of community services after stroke*

Service	9 months after stroke		18 months after stroke		1 year after stroke[a]
Home help	47%	(93)[b]	47%	(72)	19%
Meals on Wheels	26%	(93)	25%	(72)	8%
District nurse	21%	(91)	16%	(82)	19%
Bathing assistant	16%	(92)	26%	(82)	NK
Laundry service	5%	(93)	10%	(72)	1%
Lunch club	9%	(93)	18%	(72)	NK

[a] Data for 383 patients living at home in Bristol (Legh-Smith *et al.*, 1986).
[b] Figures in brackets are the numbers on which percentages are based.

59% among older patients. These differences reflect the availability of alternative support at home, and the needs of most patients were being met: no one wanted more of the Meals on Wheels service while 6 patients (8%) would have preferred to receive more of the home help service – all of these were women living alone and 5 of them were currently receiving the service. Whether patients lived alone or with others there was no relationship between supporter's sex and patient's receipt of these services, so male supporters were not receiving more of the statutory support services.

The severity of the patient's disability was not associated with use of home help and Meals on Wheels services, but 40% of the patients with moderate or severe disability had been seen by a district nurse in the preceding 4 weeks compared with only 5% of those with mild or no disability. Fewer of the patients in their sixties were receiving help from the district nurse – only 4% were, compared with 23% of older patients. However, neither use of the district nurse nor of the bathing assistant was either more or less frequent among patients who lived alone. Although nearly a quarter (22%) of women patients had been visited by the district nurse, compared with only 6% of men, this difference was not statistically significant; however, none of the men was receiving regular visits (5 or more times in the preceding 4 weeks) compared with 18% of the women. There was no difference by sex in the frequency of receiving help from the bathing assistant nor was this associated with the patient's age. Patients with female supporters were about twice as likely to receive help from a bathing assistant as were patients with male supporters (29% compared with 15%), but this difference was not statistically significant.

Bathing and cutting toenails were the activities with which the greatest number of patients needed help. Bathing was a problem for all patients with moderate or severe disability as well as for 76% of patients with mild disability. There were no differences between patients with different degrees of dependency in the proportion who received help from the bathing assistant; altogether 34% did. Clearly, bathing assistants saw only those patients who needed help to wash all over, but of those who needed help only 40% were seen. However, only 5% of patients wished they had more help from a bathing assistant and 4% felt they could have used more help from a district nurse.

Eighteen months after the stroke 30% of patients reported receiving help with their foot care from a chiropodist, but this was also the service that the largest proportion of people wanted more of. Seventeen per cent of patients wanted to see more of the chiropodist; often because the gap between treatments was judged to be too long.

The general practitioner

Among the health services, more patients were seeing their general practitioner than anyone else. At 18 months after the stroke 35% of patients reported seeing a general practitioner in the previous 4 weeks, and of the remainder 62% had seen their doctor in the last 6 months. One in ten patients said they had not seen their general practitioner at all in the 18 months since the stroke; none of the middle-class patients were in this group but it included 13% of patients classified as working-class. This difference was not statistically significant but 56% of middle-class patients reported that they had seen a general practitioner in the previous 4 weeks compared with only 29% of patients classified as working-class; this was the major difference in use of the general practitioner. Among patients living in the community the rate of consultation with the general practitioner was not associated with the patient's age, sex, household composition or home ownership. Nor was the consultation rate related to the severity of the patient's disability. However, only 24% of patients who described their health for their age as excellent or good had seen the doctor in the previous 4 weeks compared with 49% of those who rated their health as fair or poor for their age.

At the second interview patients were asked what sort of assistance their doctor had given them since the stroke and whether this had been 'very helpful', 'fairly helpful' or 'not very helpful'. Among the patients who commented on this, 38% described the doctor as having been very helpful, 43% said fairly helpful and 19% that their their general practitioner had not been helpful. Patients who had not seen their doctor in the previous month were more likely to say that he or she had not been helpful: 24% said this compared with 6% of those who had seen the doctor. The social class difference was not statistically significant, although only 32% of patients classified as working-class said the doctor had been very helpful compared with 55% of middle-class patients.

Comments from the patients indicated five main qualities which they appreciated in their doctor: providing explanation, taking blood pressure, visiting when requested, sorting out prescriptions, and helping with a practical problem such as money or housing. However, these same comments were laced with asides about it not being reasonable to expect too much and about how busy the doctors were. Patients who said the doctor was very helpful appeared to be particularly pleased about unsolicited visits. A man with chronic bronchitis noted:

She's a wonderful doctor. Nothing is too much trouble for her. She's been coming once a week up to last week. She sorts out the tablets and that. Talks to my wife more than me like, asking how I am and that.

And a patient who walked outdoors only with help was pleased because the doctor had applied for a disability allowance for the patient and also the badge that allows disabled people to park their cars in restricted areas. In general the doctor was:

Very, very helpful – she came out last week without me asking.

Among patients who described the doctor as very helpful, several expressed satisfaction that the doctor had explained problems or provided reassurance. A woman in her sixties who had mild disability recalled:

Very good, very understanding. As I say he explained the crying and the depression. But I hadn't known that. I wondered if it was because I couldn't take any more, but we [husband and patient] went to see him and he was very good.

Patients who described the doctor as fairly helpful recalled fewer specifically good incidents, but appeared to have a generally good relationship with their doctor, even if they thought there was little that could be done. Many patients at all levels of disability seemed to feel that the doctor could do little but supervise prescriptions. A woman patient with mild disability and a man with moderate disability noted, respectively:

I go once a month. No help, but prescription and she takes my blood pressure. She can't do anything else, but she's told me if I don't feel well to give her a ring. She's very good. She makes out prescriptions.

She's just been giving me tablets and that. She's only been in twice since I left hospital. She does her best, but the thing is she has too many patients. She does her best. She'll treat me if I go there. We get on well, on forename terms.

Several patients who felt the doctor had been helpful appeared to have moderated their expectations because they felt the doctor was busy. Among patients who felt the doctor had not been helpful it was clearly because of a lack of contact, rather than because they felt the doctor was unable to help. The patient might be having prescribed medicines, but a home help or relative picked it up:

Not seen her. My home help gets me a repeat of my prescription.

He never comes near nor by; he never comes. We phone him up for our prescription. No help, he never comes.

The woman who made the last comment, like the man who made the next, was housebound, living with and receiving much support from a spouse. These spouses play a role in determining use of the welfare services, as the disabled man made clear:

Gawd, if I say I'm queer it's all in the mind [wife] says. It's a waste of time calling him in. Mind over matter. Too much is mind over bloody matter, if you ask me. Haven't seen him [the GP]; he hasn't helped me. Wife goes to collect [the prescriptions] every 2 weeks.

The feeling that the general practitioner could do few specific things to help, as well as a confidence that the doctor would come if asked to, permeated responses to the question about whether patients wanted more help from their doctor. At the second interview most patients (81%) could not think of any way in which the general practitioner could help them more, 15% said they would like more help and 4% made some other comment. These proportions did not differ with the patient's sex, age, social class or household composition but, for some reason, patients with mild disability were more interested in extra help from their general practitioner: 27% of them were, compared with 6% of other patients. Possibly these patients feel somehow caught in between, neither requiring the regular support of health services nor free of disability. Most of them were looking for the reassurance of a check-up rather than other specific help with problems caused by the stroke. A woman, aged 72, living alone commented:

I think they should come and visit more often because I am one of those people who doesn't want to bother the doctor. My daughter says I should ring him, but I don't want to unless I have to.

This ambivalent feeling about bothering the doctor was a concern too for patients with obvious disability. One man who had been working before the stroke but who was, 18 months later, confined to a wheelchair felt uncertain about contacting the doctor although he wondered if more could not be done:

I've got a feeling that I don't see the doctor enough, whereas, in the hospital, I used to see Dr. Tesh more regularly. I think my doctor might come to see me more often and check my blood pressure and that. As I say, one of my troubles is that I don't seem to be getting any better and I wonder if I'm getting enough medical attention. I don't expect him to have a magic wand and I know it's a slow business, but I feel like it's a burden on the doctor and I don't think I should feel like that. I don't think he's neglecting me, but I keep believing I am ill and should be seeing more of him.

At the final interview this man still felt he could use more help from his doctor:

He's a very good doctor, but you have to prod him to come. He pops in when it suits him. He's never refused to come: he's very good.

He was one of only 7 patients (10%) who wanted more help from their general practitioner at 18 months after the stroke.

There was an attitude among several of the patients that they did not want more help from their general practitioner because they were under the hospital (still attending out-patients) or because stroke was really a problem that hospital doctors, not general practitioners, dealt with – as, during the acute phase, it was in Greenwich. A man who had returned to hospital several times since the initial stroke felt:

Well, I mean to say, I don't think he understands the case at all you see. He only goes, I suppose, on what the hospital tells him.

And another patient, who had recently been in hospital, expressed the dilemmas more generally:

It used to be with the old family doctor that he came and visited and made the diagnosis. Now, if there's anything they send you off to hospital. It's like they don't have enough time and too many patients to care for. They can only get out in the mornings. I don't blame them for not coming out at night.

Unfortunately the expectations of some of these older patients appeared to have been driven low by the experience of care that was viewed as indifferent. A housebound woman reflected on current and previous practice:

What could he do? He don't come round to see you. You don't see him unless you call for him. I've got tablets, I've got sleeping tablets. The other doctor I had used to come once a fortnight. I was sorry he left. The old one used to pop in, see if you had any complaints; if there was anything wrong you could tell him. All you get now is 'take these tablets, you'll be alright.'

Beneath the surface of apparent satisfaction with help from their general practitioners, an appreciable number of patients felt the doctor should call to see how they were even if there was nothing specific the general practitioner could do for them. Many patients appeared to value the personal relationship and the reassurance that their doctor could provide – but the 'caring interest' was often absent.

Social workers

At the second interview 22% of patients recalled the hospital social worker as having done something 'useful' for them, and this probably reflects their involvement in discharge and housing. This proportion did not vary with the patient's age, sex or initial disability, but 33% of patients who lived alone reported that the social worker had been very helpful, compared with only 12% of those who lived with others. Surprisingly, 41% of patients classified as middle-class recalled the hospital social worker giving useful help or advice, compared with only 17% of working-class patients. This picture does not necessarily reflect the proportions in which help was offered, asked for or refused, but the outcomes in terms of patient satisfaction suggest a need to investigate how much is due to more articulate middle-class patients knowing how and when to use social workers.

When patients were asked about help received during the 4 weeks before the second interview only 10% recalled a helpful contact with a social worker. There were no class-associated differences in the proportions receiving help from the social worker but 19% of patients with severe or moderate disability reported useful help in the previous 4 weeks, compared with only 5% of patients who were rated as having mild or no disability. However, it appeared that patients with the middle range of severity of disability were most likely to want more help from the social worker: only 1 of the 35 patients with disability classified as severe or normal wanted more help, compared with a quarter of the patients who had mild or moderate disability. Problems with housing and money were the main issues, and altogether 16% of patients would like to have talked over these problems with a social worker. This proportion may, in part, reflect the patient's previous experience with a social worker. There was a feeling among several patients that the social services asked about as many questions as the researcher, but with a view to doing something that never materialised. One man, for example, who had decided not to talk with the social worker, said:

Not at the moment. I was going to talk about getting a shower put in. You've got to go through them first to get to the Council. All of them came round promising everything, but it never happened. Just now [6 months after coming home] we've got the attendance allowance. They'd walk in the door, ask all your business, leave and then nothing would happen.

Altogether, a higher proportion of male patients (26%, compared with only 10% of women) wanted to see a social worker. This demand was associated with diverse problems in the transition from employment and income to retirement and pensions.

Day hospitals

Finally, among services for patients, day hospitals were available at both the main district hospitals; there were also several day centres in residential homes. The day centres and day hospitals provide different services and facilities and should not be considered to have similar functions, but they were asked about together, and 16% of patients reported that they had attended one of these day services during the 3 months before the second interview. Three-quarters of these attenders had gone weekly or more often; these proportions are similar to those reported from the Bristol study (Legh-Smith *et al.*, 1986). Attendance at the day hospital or day centre was clearly linked to the extent of dependency, increasing from none of those classified as having no disability to 16% of patients with moderate or mild disability, and 41% of patients who had severe disability.

Health and social services: services for supporters

In some respects it is difficult to disentangle services provided for patients from support for the carers, but few of the latter described themselves as receiving help from the daily social services: in the 7 days before the second interview, 13% had had help from a home help, 2% had used Meals on Wheels, 2% had gone to a lunch club and one supporter had used the laundry service for themselves. Altogether 87% of supporters had used none of these services in the previous week. The recipients of these services were, in 10 of the 12 cases, spouses of the stroke patient. Not surprisingly, no supporter under the age of 55 used any of these services, nor did any of this group say that they wanted any of these services. Indeed only one supporter who was not receiving the home help service wanted it, and none of those who were receiving a home help wanted more; none of the supporters reported wanting any of the other services that were listed.

Table 48. *Supporters' contact with services in the 9 months following the stroke*

Supporter reports:	Patient's GP (%)	District nurse (%)	Social worker (%)
No contact	46	70	57
Contact but not helpful	30	12	16
Contact and helpful	24	18	27
No. of supporters (= 100%)	95	95	95

In the first 9 months many supporters had contact with the welfare services about meeting the patient's needs. The figures in Table 48 show that more than half the supporters reported contact with the patient's general practitioner, 30% had seen a district nurse and 43% had been in touch with a social worker.

Since the district nurse generally visits to do specific tasks it is surprising that only 3 in 5 contacts were thought to be helpful. This helpful contact was usually about something to do with the patient's illness or treatment. A daughter reported:

It was to do with the drugs she's on [for cancer]. She told me not to touch this or that or it would affect me.

And a spouse who had been caring for his housebound wife for a decade said that the various district nurses had been helpful:

One in particular advised me to massage her bottom. They've all made suggestions in various ways. I like to keep them on because you're in touch with them.

Contact with the district nurse appeared to be no more or less frequent among supporters who lived with the patient, mainly because most of the supporters of patients who received help from the district nurse had contact with her or him.

During the period when patients were in hospital social workers were described as the source of help with the supporters' worries and anxieties more than any other professionals. In the interview at 1 month after the stroke 15 supporters mentioned receiving help or advice about problems with coping from the social worker, compared with only 1 supporter who mentioned rehabilitation therapists, 2 who mentioned nurses and 3 who mentioned the general practitioner. Several of the supporters who mentioned helpful advice from the social worker soon after the stroke appeared to develop close working relationships with that service. A wife, for example, reported a month after the stroke that the social worker at the hospital:

just more or less said how it was going to be, and if I had any difficulties to get in touch with them. He just said I would have to have plenty of help.

Eight months later this supporter and her husband (who described his mind as 'gone' since the stroke) were receiving regular support from the community social services:

She [the social worker] comes and talks to me one fortnight and comes to see him the next fortnight.

Many of the supporters who received help from social workers were concerned about the patient's housing, but supporters also reported receiving help about disabled badges for the car, arranging home helps and chiropodists, organising holidays, and supplying aids. Only one of the supporters mentioned that the social worker gave any financial advice. The proportion of supporters reporting help from the social worker was not associated with the hospital or ward on which the patient had been treated, but supporters of patients with mild or moderate disability 9 months after stroke were more likely to have received help – 39% said this compared with only 18% of the supporters of other patients.

Although more than half the supporters had some contact with the patient's general practitioner in the first 9 months after the stroke, only a quarter of them described a contact in which the assistance, instruction or advice was regarded as helpful. The proportion of supporters who reported contact was not linked to the severity of the patient's disability, but spouses were more likely than other relatives to have contact (79% compared with 41%) and 44% of spouses described a helpful contact compared with 14% of other relatives.

The patient's general practitioner was reported as making the contacts with supporters 'helpful' by advising on the patient's diet, medicines and coping with depression, by providing reassurance about progress, about the results of tests and about the doctor's availability, and by helping with some practical tasks such as obtaining disabled badges or a letter to the housing department.

Inevitably, some of these contacts with the doctor responded to the supporter's concerns as well as coping with the patient's needs. In many cases the general practitioner was likely to know the supporter well. Among the supporters seen 18 months after the stroke 49% had the same general practitioner as the patient, 3% had a different doctor in the same practice, 44% identified a general practitioner in another practice and 1% had a general practitioner but did not specify where. Three per cent of supporters said they had no general practitioner. At the third interview supporters were asked if they had seen their own general practitioner for themselves to discuss any difficulty caused by the patient's stroke. Of these supporters only one-fifth said they had discussed problems with their own doctor; 6 supporters (8% of all) felt this contact had been very helpful, 4 that it had been fairly helpful and 4 that it was not helpful. Of these 14 supporters who had spoken with their doctor about themselves, 12 were women; and 11 had the same doctor as the patient.

Finally, supporters were asked at both the second and third interviews whether there were any people in the health service or from social services who they felt should have helped more or who should currently be helping them more. At the second interview 30% of supporters identified such a person, as did 31% of supporters at the third interview. There was some continuity in these responses, insofar as 56% of carers who wanted more help 9 months after the stroke also indicated this at 18 months after the stroke. In general, there was no common characteristic among the supporters who wanted more help – on neither occasion were the proportions who wanted more help related to the age or sex of the patients, or to the severity of the patient's disability; nor was the relationship of the supporter to the patient, the supporter's sex, self-rated health or whether he or she was living with the patient a distinguishing characteristic; and experience of previous contacts with their own general practitioner, district nurse or social worker did not appear to make much difference. However, supporters who had seen the patient's general practitioner were more likely to want further help – 43% said this compared with 19% of other supporters.

On the whole, demand for more help – almost always to help the patient, and, therefore, indirectly the supporter – was tied to specific problems. The focus was heavily on the need for the social services, social workers and the Department of Social Security to assist with housing for the patient, money and holidays. Several of the supporters felt they were given little help in the difficult job of sorting out a new home for the patient. The sister of a severely disabled woman, in her sixties, who spent almost a year in hospital said:

They keep sending us lists of nursing homes. They are passing the buck. They should sort out the nursing home for us, then we could go and look at it. The social worker should be doing a lot more in as much as finding something decent.

At the second interview 5 of the supporters commented on the lack of help from the patient's general practitioner, mainly in terms of a failure to keep in touch with the patient.

At the third interview supporters expressed a more general dismay with the way events had turned out. Their reference to the welfare services was more in the nature of feeling that support could have been better, even if the outcomes might not have been very different. Two-thirds of the comments were directed to inadequacies in these services, particularly to a lack of continuing support from social workers after the patient came home from hospital. Neither patients nor supporters appeared to receive much counselling in accommodating to their changed circumstances.

Even in the context of relatively high levels of support for patients from community services, a small number of supporters felt that they and the patient had been neglected since the stroke. The wife of a man in his sixties with mild residual disability felt that 'anybody' could have helped more:

No one has come near us. This is what has made me so bitter, so cross. We've had to fight our way through it. We've got bitter memories about [the hospital]; it was sink or swim. Nobody ever comes to see if he's alright. They're special cases, stroke cases, but they've never shown an interest.

Patients with stroke also present complex cases, with needs that cross the whole spectrum of provision in the health and social services. Several of the supporters commented that, even after 18 months, they felt they did not know about services or about benefits that existed.

SUMMARY

Leaving hospital Patients who were more severely disabled stayed in hospital for longer. However, none of the patients who had lived at home with their spouse before the stroke remained in hospital for 9 months or more, compared with 14% of patients from other households. Patients who lived alone were not more likely to stay in hospital longer, nor was the patient's duration of stay associated with the type of accommodation they had lived in before the stroke. Few patients reported problems with arrangements for leaving hospital.

Home Over the 18 months after the stroke nearly a third of the patients moved house. Among survivors at the third interview 10% had moved into sheltered housing – none of these people were previously owner-occupiers. A further 10% of patients had moved permanently into institutional care. Only 3% of the patients who had shared a home with their spouse before the stroke went into institutional care compared with

20% of patients who had been living alone in the community before the stroke. Patients who remained moderately or severely disabled 18 months after the stroke were more likely to have moved into institutional care. Both patients and supporters felt that the housing of patients with moderate or severe disability was less suitable than that of other survivors. In particular, the supporters of these more disabled patients were unhappy about accommodation in a hospital or nursing home. Half the patients reported having had some adaptations made to their home or some aids put in, and most found these aids or adaptations useful, even 18 months after the stroke.

Support in the community   The main source of help and support is the patient's family. At 18 months after the stroke half the patients living in the community, particularly women and those aged 80 or over, were living alone; 71% of these patients said they received most of their help and support from their children and 16% said this came from siblings. Altogether only 6% of survivors described someone other than family or friends as having been the main source of help and support since the stroke, but for different kinds of support – with mobility and self-care, with emotional and social support – spouses (especially for men) generally followed by children were mentioned most often.

Patients received more help from formal services for looking after themselves (district nurses, bathing assistants, chiropodists) than for getting about. One in 7 of the patients felt they needed more help to get about; a slightly lower proportion wanted more help with self-care. Although there was some disappointment about a lack of help, or interest, from diverse sources, most people did not expect more help from family, neighbours or anyone else.

Supporters, too, received most of their support from family, but at 18 months after the stroke 28% of supporters identified someone from their family or friends they felt could have helped more – mainly children of the patient. A third of supporters felt that no one in particular had given them any practical support, but this proportion fell with increasing disability of the patient. The sons and daughters of the patients were most likely to feel that family and friends, particularly their brothers and sisters, should have given more help.

Help from the health and social services   Among patients there was marked continuity in use of community services between 9 and 18 months after the stroke.

In the longer-term half the patients were receiving the home help service and a quarter had Meals on Wheels. Three-quarters or more of these recipients lived alone. Use was not associated with severity of the disability, nor did male supporters receive more of these statutory services to help them. The district nurse was the only service investigated in which use was related clearly to the severity of the patient's disability. Bathing and cutting toenails were personal services with which about one-third of patients received help, and chiropody was the service that the largest proportion wanted more of.

A third of patients reported seeing their general practitioner in the 4 weeks before the final interview. The proportion was higher among middle-class patients, but not associated with severity of disability. At 9 months after the stroke over a third of the patients described their general practitioner as having been very helpful since the stroke; 'caring interest' rather than technical skill was regarded as missing by some patients. More than half the middle-class patients described their doctor as very helpful compared with only a third of working-class patients, but the difference was not significant. It also appeared that middle-class patients found the help of social workers more useful than did those classified as working-class. One in 6 patients, but 1 in 4 men, wanted to talk over some problem with a social worker, principally one to do with housing or money.

The supporter's general practitioner was the same as the patient's in half the cases, but at 18 months after the stroke only a fifth of supporters said they had seen the general practitioner for themselves to discuss any problem caused by the stroke. In the community supporters received relatively little help from health and social services, although one-third of supporters felt they could have used more help and advice – again mainly about housing, holiday breaks and money.

In the longer-term there was some disappointment among supporters about the lack of continuity in social work support after the patient came home from hospital.

CHAPTER SEVEN

The effects of stroke on social, family and personal life

The recognition and treatment of the emotional and social consequences of stroke is both difficult and important. These aspects have been sadly neglected although they probably constitute the most problematic elements in rehabilitation, and cause most distress to the patient's family. As Newman (1984) has indicated, those concerned with the processes of recovery and rehabilitation need to look at both the family and the wider social context if they are to be successful at reintegrating stroke patients in the community. The emphasis in everyday life is upon the handicap resulting from the stroke, and that is the focus of this chapter. In particular, the analyses will concentrate on aspects of change following the stroke – in social and domestic activities, mood and emotions, family relationships and specifically the relationship between the patient and supporter.

Housework

Before the stroke, five-sixths of the patients were doing some housework, but this is one activity that most reduce without discrimination by sex or age. Altogether four-fifths of patients were doing less than they had before the stroke. The pattern of changes in scores for housework activities before and after the stroke is shown in Table 49, which demonstrates that most of the reduction has occurred by 9 months after the stroke. Among survivors to 18 months after stroke, the average scores for housework (see Appendix) fell from 16.3 before the stroke to 12.0 at 9 months and to 10.9 at 18 months. The severity of disability 1 month after the stroke was not related consistently to the extent of the decline in performance of housework.

The views of patients about how much housework they were doing compared with before the stroke followed measured change closely.

Table 49. *Changes in patients' housework scores with time after the stroke*

Change	T0 to T2[a] (%)	T2 to T3 (%)	T0 to T3 (%)
+7 to 9	1	0	0
+4 to 6	2	2	1
+1 to 3	8	16	3
0	15	40	14
−1 to 3	18	29	22
−4 to 6	29	9	22
−7 to 9	11	3	20
−10 to 12	6	0	11
−13 to 15	6	1	4
−16 to 18	4	0	3
No. of patients (=100%)	109	92	92

[a] T0, before the stroke; T2, 9 months after the stroke; T3, 18 months after the stroke.

Altogether half the patients felt they were doing much less than before the stroke, and a quarter that they were doing slightly less. The proportion of patients who said they were doing much less increased from 8% of patients who were actually doing as much or more than they had before the stroke to 92% of those whose performance had fallen by 10 or more points. The views of patients and supporters about how much less the patient was doing agreed in two-thirds of the cases.

Participation in all the household activities fell sharply after the stroke. The proportion of patients who said that in the 3 months preceding the interview they had done any of the different activities is shown in Table 50, which compares life before the stroke with that 18 months later. The scale of change is illustrated in the last column of Table 50 as the proportion of patients who before the stroke did the activity regularly ('most days' for cooking and washing up, 'weekly' for the others) but at 18 months after the stroke had not done it at all in the previous 3 months.

At 18 months after the stroke patients with severe disability were not doing less housework than those with moderate disability, but both groups (average housework score 6.5) were doing a lot less than patients with mild disability (average score 11.5) and those with no measured dependency on the Barthel index (average score 17.0). Although people living alone were no more or less disabled than other patients they were doing more housework themselves, with an average score of 12.8 compared with 9.3 for patients living with others. As expected the sex difference

Table 50. *Change in patients' housework activities from before the stroke to 18 months after the stroke*

| Housework activities | Proportion reporting doing activity in the previous 3 months[a] | | Proportion reducing from 'regular' to 'never' (%) |
	Before stroke (%)	18 months after stroke (%)	
Prepare main meals	60	35	24
Washing up	84	55	30
Wash clothes	54	29	24
Light housework	71	39	28
Heavy housework	45	9	15
Local shopping	61	30	24

[a] Data for 92 patients interviewed at both 1 and 18 months after the stroke.

was maintained, with men doing less than women (average scores 8.6 and 12.4 respectively). There was also a trend for less housework activity with increasing age: the proportion of patients scoring 15 or more points fell from 50% of those aged 60–69 to only 13% of those aged 80 or over. There was no association with social class.

The relatively low level of housework activity at 18 months after the stroke was regarded by a majority of patients as causing them 'no problem' – someone else did it. Altogether 61% of patients felt that the housework did not cause them a problem; this was said by 83% of men but by only 47% of women patients. Twelve per cent of supporters regarded the patient's housework as a 'great problem', either because it was a struggle for them to do it themselves or because they were not satisfied with the quality of the work done by others.

Social activities

Change over time

Patients were not spending the time released from housework by being more socially active, at least not as assessed in this study. Nor, on the whole, were they very much less active after the stroke: the average score for the social activities that were investigated (see Appendix) was 13.0 for life before the stroke, 11.8 at 9 months and 12.0 at 18 months after the

Table 51. *Changes in patients' social activities scores with time after the stroke*

Change	T0 to T2[a]	T2 to T3	T0 to T3
	%	%	%
+7 or more	0	0	0
+5 to 6	1	1	1
+3 to 4	3	8	6
+1 to 2	14	25	15
0	29	36	21
−1 to 2	29	25	29
−3 to 4	17	3	19
−5 to 6	2	2	6
−7 or less	5	0	3
No. of patients (=100%)	101	88	90

[a] T0, before the stroke; T2, 9 months after the stroke; T3, 18 months after the stroke.

stroke. The relative constancy of these scores masks considerable changes following the stroke, and altogether social activities declined for more than half the patients, as shown in Table 51.

There was no difference in the extent of change over time associated with the patient's sex, marital status or social class, but younger patients made greater reductions in their social activity: for example the score for patients aged 60–74 fell by an average of 2.0 compared with a drop of 0.4 among patients aged 75 and over. Altogether two-thirds of younger patients reduced their activities compared with less than half the patients aged 75 or over. This difference was, in large part, because patients who were more socially active before the stroke subsequently reduced their activities more than did the less active patients: the trend went from an increase in score, from before the stroke to 18 months later, of 0.5 among patients who scored 11 or less for life before the stroke, to a decrease of 3.7 among patients who were active enough to score 16 or more points for life before the stroke. Finally, patients with more severe disability gave up more activities, but the differences were not statistically significant: the activities of patients who had no disability after the stroke fell by 0.3, compared with a decrease of 1.7 for patients who were classified as having severe disability 1 month after the stroke.

The relatively weak relationship between changes in physical disability and social activity suggests that some patients curtail their lives in excess of their physical limitations due, for example, to fear, poor advice, lack of social support, poor self-image or low morale. Several authors have specifically considered the effects of depression on social activities, indicating that patients who are depressed after a stroke are likely to reduce their social activities to a greater extent (Feibel and Springer, 1982; Robinson *et al.*, 1985). However, the nature of these studies does not permit a distinction to be made between changes in mental state that are a cause, consequence or co-occurrence of changes in social activity. Among patients in Greenwich the extent of social activities before the stroke was not associated with scores for emotional distress 1 month after the stroke. But equally the scores for emotional distress 1 month after the stroke were not associated either with change in scores for social activity from before the stroke to 18 months later, or with the level of social activity 18 months after the stroke. So it appears that depression (Ebrahim *et al.* (1986) argue that among stroke patients the measure of emotional distress is a valid indicator of depressed mood) is not a useful predictor of reduced social activities.

This lack of a relationship may be due to the relatively low levels of social activity before the stroke and consequently to the relatively small scope for reduction in social activities. There is also the usual difficulty that in different studies the various main variables have been assessed using different methods. The social activities index may not be sensitive to the range and frequency of changes in daily social contacts and leisure interests. Certainly, patients with higher levels of emotional distress at 18 months after the stroke were more likely to view themselves as socialising much less since the stroke: the proportion reporting this increased from 13% of the patients rated as exhibiting no distress to 64% of those who responded positively to five or more of the items on the measure of emotional distress. However, this relationship was not evident when level of distress 1 month after the stroke was considered in relation to the patient's assessment of change 18 months after the stroke. The paths of cause and effect between these variables thus require further investigation.

Altogether 34% of patients reported that they were, 18 months after the stroke, doing things socially with other people 'much less'. The proportion rose from 19% among those whose measured participation had actually increased, up to 63% of those whose social activities score had fallen by 5 or more points. However, 41% of the patients whose scores showed them to be doing as much or more than before the stroke, also felt they were doing less socially. This may be true insofar as the range of frequencies within the categories of response was wide. The documentation of handicap after stroke demands improvements, particularly in the assessment of social activity and changes in functioning over time.

There were two specific activities for which the frequency of participation was significantly reduced. At 18 months after the stroke only 15% of patients reported that they had been on a day trip or an outing in the previous 3 months, whereas 36% of them had reported this as happening during the 3 months before their stroke. Secondly, the proportion of patients who said they went out to visit family or friends at least once a week fell from 40% for life before the stroke to 16% at 18 months later. So, as Labi and colleagues (1980) found in an American community population, there is, not surprisingly, greater difficulty resuming activities outside the home. The decline in visiting family among patients in Greenwich was somewhat compensated for by an increase in family or friends visiting the patients: 78% of patients reported visits every week or more often at 18 months after the stroke compared with 71% who had reported this for the 3 months before their stroke – but the difference was not significant. It was noted in Chapter 2 that the patients' social lives before the stroke were dominated by contacts with family. This was equally so at the third interview. The average score for 'family contacts' was unchanged over the 18 months after the stroke. And although there were patients whose contacts increased (17% of all patients) and decreased (40%), these changes were not associated with the patient's sex, age, social class, marital status or the severity of disability at 1 month after the stroke.

The patients' supporters were asked for their assessments about how the patients' social, leisure and family involvement had changed from before the stroke to 18 months later. The responses are shown in Table 52. Patients and supporters agreed over the extent of change in the patients' socialising in only 40% of cases. Supporters tended to categorise patients with small declines in measured activity as doing 'much less'; for example, among patients whose measured change was an increase of 1–4 points on the social activities index, 39% of supporters said the patient was doing much less, as did 48% of the supporters of patients with a fall in score of 1–4 points. These figures may say as much about the supporters as the patients. Spouses were more likely to observe that the patient was doing much less socially – 54% of them said this compared with 27% of other relatives. However, there was no association in general between the supporter's view and the sex or age of the patient, nor with whether the supporter lived with the patient.

The views of supporters afford another perspective from which to consider the relationship between physical disability or emotional distress and subsequent changes in social activity. The supporters' assessments show a clear and consistent pattern: patients with little or no emotional

Table 52. *Supporters' assessments of changes in patient's social and family involvement*

Compared with before stroke patient now does:	Show interest in family or friends (%)	Keep busy doing things (%)	Take part in conversations (%)	Do things socially with other people (%)
Much less	26	49	26	44
Slightly less	21	27	15	16
No change	48	21	52	40
More	5	3	7	0
No. of supporters (= 100%)	75	75	73	75

Table 53. *Patient's physical and emotional condition 1 month after the stroke related to supporters' assessments of changes in patients' social behaviour*

Supporters' views comparing before the stroke and 18 months later[a]	Emotional distress score 1 month after stroke		Barthel (disability) rating 1 month after stroke	
	0–2 (%)	3+ (%)	Mild/normal (%)	Moderate/severe (%)
Shows interest in family or friends	8	41	23	28
Keeps busy doing things	28	76	38	61
Takes part in conversations	8	34	18	34
Does things socially with other people	33	55	28	61
No. of patients (= 100%)	36	30	39	36

[a] Proportion of patients described as doing 'much less'.

distress at 1 month after the stroke were generally less likely to be described by their supporters as doing 'much less' of the different activities. This is shown in Table 53, which also indicates a weaker pattern of links between the patient's disability 1 month after the stroke, and the supporter's assessment 18 months after the stroke of changes in the patient's social behaviour.

Eighteen months after the stroke

The patient's involvement in social activities 18 months after the stroke was, as for housework, not very different for patients with severe or moderate disability. However the average score for these patients (10.5) was lower than that for patients with mild disability (12.4) or with no disability (13.9). This relationship between physical disability and social activities at one point in time was also found for life before the stroke. Christie (1982) argues, from his study in Melbourne, Australia, that residual weakness is not a necessary or sufficient cause of handicap, but patients in Greenwich were generally doing so few of the activities investigated that those with moderate or severe disability appeared seldom to go out for social contacts; only 27% of them reported that they had been out to visit family or friends in the previous 3 months, compared with 78% of patients who had mild or no disability. There was no difference with degree of residual disability in the receipt of visits from family or friends. A similar pattern emerged that people with higher levels of emotional distress 18 months after the stroke were engaged in fewer social activities (although the correlation was relatively unimpressive: $r = 0.14$). As was the case with disability, the main difference was that half the patients with scores of 3 or more on the emotional distress scale had not been out to visit family or friends in the previous 3 months compared with a quarter of the patients who were less distressed.

At a given point in time emotional distress and social activities were thus related. However, it seems as plausible to argue that social contacts, particularly with family, influence self-image and morale, as it is to suggest that feelings of emotional distress result in a reduction in social activities. There were no significant associations between the total social activities score and the patient's sex, marital status or social class, but those patients who were aged 80 or over were doing less: they had an average social activities score of 10.7 compared with an average score of 12.5 for younger patients.

As was the case with housework, only 12% of patients felt that doing things socially, with other people, caused them a 'great problem'; 28% said it caused 'some problem' and 60% that it was 'no problem'. Patients who were doing more appeared less likely to find it a problem: only 18% of patients who scored 16 or more said social contacts were a problem, compared with 44% of those who were less socially active – but the difference was not significant. Thus older patients, although they were doing less, were not more likely to describe social contact with other people as a problem. People who had more severe disability 1 month after the stroke were more likely, 18 months later, to report that doing things socially was a problem, this proportion increasing from 25% of patients with no measured disability to 54% of those with severe disability. Viewing social life as a problem was not associated with social class or sex. Altogether, at the third interview, a quarter of the patients said that they wished they saw more of their family and friends.

Many patients apparently had little interest in social involvement with others. At 9 months after the stroke 38% of patients said that in the previous few months they had not wanted to get together socially with other people and 40% said they had wanted this 'just a little'. Therefore the group of patients who at the third interview said that doing things socially caused no problem includes many who do not express a need for much social contact or who view the prospect of contact as uninviting. Many patients appear to have led most of their lives between work and home, or work at home. A married man confined to his wheelchair who found social life was no problem said:

Well, as I said, I've no friends that sort of way. If you don't have anything like it in the beginning, you don't miss it or anything after. I never used to go out of a night-time; pubs and drinking and that was out of my line. When I was at work I used to come home, shut the door, make something to eat and then lie on the bed to listen to the wireless.

And a woman with eight children who also found little social life no problem commented:

I never was a one – I was always indoors with having children and that.

For other patients a lack of company was preferred. A woman noted that:

When you've got troubles of your own, you don't really want to. That's all people seem to talk about – their problems. And I worry about other people.

Another woman expressed similar feelings:

I don't like a lot of people around me. I don't like company with a lot of people. My sister is bad enough, lousy with it. But all she comes with are her moans – she's the only widow in the world.

Among the patients who found mixing socially a problem, this was almost always attributable to some consequence of the stroke. A man who had lost confidence in himself since the stroke, and who tended to choke when eating, went to a social club:

But how would you feel there with ten women, old, who can't speak and you're the only man. Don't like it at all, but it gives [wife] a break.

He described mixing socially as a great problem, but mainly because of the difficulty with eating. A woman who also felt that mixing socially was a great problem said:

I'm very embarrassed that I can't talk and I can't walk to go anywhere.

In general, as discussed later in this chapter, patients with speech problems found it much more difficult to mix with others. Patients with significant loss of physical ability but without speech problems appeared to accommodate quite well to reduced activity: only 10% of them described doing things socially with other people as a great problem. One man, whose life had changed from being the chairman of a voluntary organisation with meetings four nights a week to long-term stays in hospital and mobility only in a wheelchair, explained:

I don't do anything. It doesn't bother me much, but I'm slipping, aren't I? I used to chair meetings and control them, but that's gone now.

And a woman who went out a lot with family and friends before the stroke commented:

I like doing things with other people, but I've come to terms with it, that anything I can't do now is due to my illness.

However, one patient who also felt social life was 'some problem' identified a specific factor confounding the difficulties caused by the stroke:

Because of my handicap I suppose it's got to be a bit of a problem. But you're putting the cart before the horse; you've got to see it in terms of your age – as you get older people don't want to talk with you so much.

Hobbies

Before the stroke the patients' principal leisure interests were carried out in the home. Between the stroke and 18 months later patients' hobbies changed considerably; a quarter of those who reported a hobby at the time of the stroke reported none 18 months later – a proportion that was not associated with the patient's sex or social class, nor with the severity of disability. There was no change in the high proportion (seven-eighths) of patients who reported watching television, but among survivors 18 months after the stroke the proportion who listened to the radio fell from 70% to 52% (contrary to the finding in the Manchester study: Brockle-hurst *et al.*, 1978*a*), and the proportion of patients who said they read newspapers, books or magazines fell from 93% to 74%. Patients had problems concentrating or taking an interest in old hobbies. A woman with no disability said:

I used to love the radio, but I don't now. Same as reading. I used to love it but I can't get any interest now.

And another woman who had knitted blankets and designed toys for charities felt:

I've had enough with the toys. I just feel as though I can't concentrate on it.

For the same reasons patients reduced the quality or quantity of their hobbies. A man whose comfortable home was lined with books commented:

I can read a bit, not as much as I'd like. I can't hold my concentration for long enough; if it's a big book it seems to pall on me.

Several patients mentioned that their eyesight was worse after the stroke, dictating a loss in their leisure pursuits. A woman who had moved into a residential home noted:

My eyes have deteriorated a lot. I can't see to knit or read the paper.

And a woman who lived alone in sheltered housing had reduced her hobbies because her eyesight was now poor:

I'm hurt, because I've lost my sight. I used to do a lot of sewing – covers and things for the children.

Patients also reduced or limited their hobbies for the more obvious physical reasons that they 'couldn't hold the wool' or 'can't get the grip in that right hand'.

In comparison with before the stroke only half as many patients mentioned that they were knitting, sewing or crocheting and no one mentioned gardening. Two of the patients who had been enthusiastic gardeners before the stroke commented that they had given up: in one case because 'I can't keep my balance, can't stoop' and in the other case because the plants were now kept indoors. The proportions of patients who mentioned reading and crosswords or games as a hobby doubled (to 4 and 2 out of 10 respectively) and 1 in 8 of the patients listed writing, drawing or some artistic activity as a hobby. Clearly their hobbies were now even more indoor-based than before the stroke; only 3 patients mentioned any active interest, including a woman who walked down to Greenwich pier to do her knitting.

The proportion of patients who mentioned a hobby had therefore changed little (it was 57%), but the hobbies were nearly all chair-based.

Emotional distress

Three studies, using different methods, appear to agree that at any time up to a third of stroke survivors may be depressed during the year after the stroke. Brocklehurst and colleagues (1978a) followed their patients at 6-week intervals for 1 year. Depression was assessed by the research interviewer on a 5-point scale ('very cheerful' to 'very depressed'). Altogether the results indicated that 29% of patients suffered from depression during most of the illness, and in 3% this seemed to be very severe. One in five of the survivors at 1 year were not initially depressed but became so during the year. In a study of all hospitalised stroke patients in one community (Rochester, New York) depression was determined by nurses' observation of patient mood, behaviour and somatic complaints; at 6 months after the stroke 26% of patients were rated as depressed (Feibel and Springer, 1982). Results from the Frenchay stroke study (Wade, 1984), in which depression was assessed systematically using the Wakefield scale, indicate that at the end of the first year 31–41% of survivors were depressed (the figure depends on the categorisation of confused, dysphasic and other patients who cannot be assessed). From his review of this literature House (1987) has estimated that depression may be almost twice as common among patients in the first year after stroke as among the normal elderly population; but the studies available make it difficult to conclude that depression is more common among patients after stroke than among older people with other physical illnesses.

Emotional distress was assessed, in Greenwich, with the Nottingham Health Profile, yielding a score which may provide some indication of depression (Ebrahim et al., 1986). There was very little change in average scores over time and, as Table 54 shows, relatively small changes for individual patients between the interviews. None of the standard variables – sex, age, social class, marital status, living alone – were associated with changes in levels of emotional distress. And although it has been suggested that depression is more common among patients with damage to the left hemisphere of the brain (Robinson and Price, 1982), there was no association among the patients in Greenwich between side of the stroke and score, or change in scores, on the measure of emotional distress.

Patients tended to remain in broadly the same degree of distress, so that

Table 54. *Changes in patients' scores for emotional distress with time after the stroke*

Change	T1 to T2[a] (%)	T2 to T3 (%)	T1 to T3 (%)
+4 or more	7	3	4
+3	6	4	3
+2	1	6	7
+1	19	21	17
0	26	26	31
−1	19	18	21
−2	15	8	10
−3	6	13	4
−4 or less	1	1	3
No. of patients (= 100%)	88	72	71

[a] T1, 1 month after the stroke; T2, 9 months after the stroke; T3, 18 months after the stroke.

patients who were distressed at the first interview were also likely to be distressed at the third interview ($r = 0.71$): among those who scored 3 or more at the first interview, 76% scored 3 or more at the third interview; among those who scored 2 or fewer at the first interview, 84% scored 2 or fewer at the third interview. The relative stability of the scores appears to support the argument that the profile reflects aspects of a depressive illness rather than representing only a reaction of adjustment to the stroke. Other studies of depression among stroke patients have similarly reported that its prevalence is fairly constant over the first year or two after the stroke (House, 1987).

Eighteen months after the stroke the only measure of disability that was significantly related to the patient's emotional distress was level of disability at that time: the average score for patients with moderate or severe disability was 3.7, compared with 2.3 for those with mild or no disability. Few characteristics have been identified that are clearly associated with depression (Robinson and Price, 1982; Feibel and Springer, 1982). In Greenwich, the distress score was not related to the patient's marital status, age, sex, initial disability or, in general, to the patient's social class; however, the proportion scoring at the high level of 4.0 or more was only 12% of middle-class patients, compared with 41% of those classified as working-class. (Is this an instance of 'denial' among middle-class patients?) Altogether, at 18 months after the stroke 35% of patients agreed with the statement 'I wake up feeling depressed', while 58% of patients acknowledged 'I feel frustrated with my situation' and 39% said they had weeping spells. None of these responses was related to the age, sex or social class of the patient.

The main differences on specific items of the emotional distress measure (see Appendix) were firstly that men more often agreed with the items reflecting loss of mastery: 25% of men but only 7% of women said they felt they were losing control; and 36% of men compared with 9% of women reported that they lost their temper easily. Secondly, more disabled patients were particularly likely to agree with the items that appear to represent low morale: 57% of those with moderate or severe disability agreed that things were getting them down, compared with 31% of patients who were rated, 18 months after the stroke, as having mild or no disability; the corresponding proportions for 'I feel that life is not worth living' were 38% and 12%; and for 'I wake up feeling depressed' the figures were 57% and 25%. There are, therefore, differences in the patient's emotional response to the stroke associated with aspects of physical disability and gender. It is also evident that even 18 months after the stroke a high proportion of patients suffer serious distress and disorders of mood; more than one-third of the patients responded positively to four or more items on the measure of emotional distress. There are major variations between studies in rates of pharmacological treatment (e.g. Coughlan and Humphrey, 1982: cf. Robinson and Price, 1982), and House (1987) argues the need to give more attention to physical methods of treatment, as well as to rehabilitation, reassurance and advice for the patient and family. Naturally a prerequisite for more active treatment of persisting emotional distress in stroke patients is increased awareness and improved assessment by doctors in the community (Newman, 1984; Goldberg, 1985; Warlow *et al.*, 1987).

Social isolation

The degree of social isolation among patients appeared to change very little over time after the stroke: after 18 months, one-third of scores were slightly higher, one-third slightly lower and one-third the same as they had been a month after the stroke. None of the variables investigated was related to change over time, except that feelings of social isolation declined for 41% of women but for only 15% of men.

Responses to individual items in the profile reveal high levels of isolation and discomfort among certain groups, and emphasise the high risk of social isolation following the stroke (Isaacs *et al.*, 1976; Labi *et al.*, 1980). Over half the male survivors agreed with a statement 'I feel I am a burden to people' compared with just over a quarter of the women; this is probably attributable in part to the higher proportion of men who live in a household with other people. And contrary to the suggestion that middle-class people might deny their feelings, 60% of them agreed with the statement 'I feel lonely' at 18 months after the stroke, compared with 25% of patients classified as working-class. However, the average score on the social isolation index of 1.2 was not related to social class, sex, age or severity of disability at 18 months after stroke.

Stigma

Few of the patients said that they felt generally socially ostracised or discriminated against because of the stroke, although at 9 months after the stroke 20% of patients agreed with the statement 'I feel that other people are uncomfortable with me'. By the third interview this proportion had fallen to 4%, while 10% of patients agreed that 'I feel other people treat me like an inferior person' and 7% felt that 'Other people would prefer to avoid me'. Labi and colleagues (1980) suggested that there may be social differences in sensitivity to loss of social status and questioned whether stroke might have a greater effect, in this respect, on women. There were no sex differences in the findings of this study but 27% of middle-class patients compared with only 6% of patients classified as working-class agreed that 'Other people treat me like an inferior person'.

Two patients (3%) agreed with all three statements and 88% agreed with none, indicating a low level of perceived stigma. However, at 18 months after the stroke 18% of patients reported feeling that since their illness other people had treated them differently. This different treatment was equally shared between experience that made living with the stroke easier and those that made it harder. Many patients volunteered that family and friends had been kind and considerate, as they always were, but several patients sensed a change. A woman with no disability felt:

People have been kinder, because they know I've been ill, whereas before you stood on your own feet, and didn't have to have anybody.

And another woman attributed improved relations with her youngest daughter to having to overcome the difficulties caused by the stroke. She felt her daughter showed:

More respect in a way, more concern.

There were relatively few patients who described experiences that are often suggested as following stroke. A man who had worked as a journalist felt that everyone treated him somewhat differently following the stroke:

... even in the hospital. They talk over you, past you. One day on ward round sister says to Dr Moriarty 'He's quite intelligent you know.' There's a tendency with everyone who's had a stroke to think you're deaf and stupid and ignore you. They talk as if you are not there.

And a woman described how her husband had embarrassed her:

When I went up Holm Lane, and we called in the florists, and I gave him a £5 note, and he treated me as if I was an imbecile, as if I was stone deaf.

However, these negative experiences were recalled by fewer than 1 in 10 of the patients. This may be because patients simply did not notice, or because events had occurred shortly after the stroke, or because most patients spent little time in social company where the experience of discrimination might occur. It seems probable also that patients make fairly generous allowances for changes in the behaviour of others, and in general they tend not to observe, or at least not to report, negative consequences of the stroke – certainly not as much as the supporters.

The patient as a person

One issue that patients and supporters appeared to view quite differently was change in the patient's personality. Altogether 45% of patients but 62% of supporters felt that the patient had changed as a person in the 18 months following the stroke. When the patient felt changed as a person, in 70% of cases supporters agreed; but when the patient denied a change in personality 55% of supporters disagreed.

The proportion of patients and supporters who identified a change in the patient's personality was not associated with the patient's age, sex, social class or the severity of the disability. Among supporters, perception of change was not significantly related to their sex, although 67% of women supporters saw change while only 47% of male supporters did. Supporters who lived with the patient were no more likely to have noticed change in the patient as a person than those who did not. However, while accepting that the small numbers involved mean the difference was not statistically significant, it is interesting that when the patients were men 77% of those who lived with them observed a change in mood or personality whereas only 50% of the supporters who lived with women patients felt that they had changed. It is not easy to disentangle whether this is a product of the patient's sex or the supporter's sex, or both. (There was no difference between men and women supporting women patients, but the number of men supporting male patients is too small for cross-analysis.) Among the supporters who lived with patients, 38% of male supporters compared with 73% of female supporters observed a change in the patient's personality.

These changes, whether viewed by patients or supporters, were generally negative. Patients often saw themselves as becoming miserable; a man with moderate disability who lived with his wife said:

I'm always miserable. I'm never happy unless I'm miserable.

And a woman with mild disability living alone described herself as:

Socially I'm the most miserable person alive lately. I try not to be, but even my grandchildren ... I was praying they would go and yet I love them so much.

Another man with mild disability living with his wife felt he had become a:

Bloody misery mate, to everyone around me. My personality's changed since I had the stroke. I know that. Now you might be complaining about things that never bothered you before, and all the things I'm talking about now are trivialities, not really worth moaning about.

Patients also viewed themselves as being irritable. A woman with mild disability living with siblings saw herself:

Flaring up over little things. I hate people to contradict me when I know I'm right. It used to be water off a duck's back, but not now. I'm much more testy now.

And a man with mild disability who lived with his wife said:

I get a bit aereated. I can't help it. I get frustrated. I don't know how she sticks me sometimes. Some wives would have chucked me out. I go mad, like when I can't do things myself.

A woman with mild disability who lived alone assessed the change in herself:

I can only assume that it's because I want to be as I was before that I get so bad tempered, like I was with the district nurse this morning. I know there are a lot of people worse than I am. I'm an awkward person and demanding. I cry and I'm very upset. I'm so restless all the time.

Patients recognised too that they felt frustrated. As two men with moderate and mild disability respectively noted:

Well, sometimes I think I am [changed] by getting frustrated, and I get depressed. Mornings are a job getting up. I feel the world is not worth facing. I feel inadequate. I want to do things – go into the workshop and mess about.

Well, I can't really say I have changed, but I moan to myself that I can't get about. The only thing I get a kick out of and that's dreams of walking – I've had two or three of those. Of course when I wake up I'm disillusioned then that I can't. I feel a bit helpless now that I can't get about and that.

Supporters tended to identify a wider range of changes in the patient as a person. Four supporters described an improvement, as they saw it, in the patient: being more tolerant, caring or appreciative. The others identified the patients as quieter, more withdrawn, irritable, aggressive and depressed. Some supporters saw the change as all-embracing. The wife of a mildly disabled man, who had a speech problem, said:

He's just not my George, not as he was. His nature has completely changed. You can't get through to him. He's the reverse of what he was.

The wife of another patient who had mild residual disability (although getting about was a great effort) felt that:

He's different to what he was before. He doesn't think of the little things he did before. He was very affectionate; he's not so loving as he was before.

And, finally, the son of a housebound patient observed:

General deterioration. She used to do things for herself, take pride in her clothes, do a bit of painting. Now all her interest in life is gone. She keeps praying to die.

To put some perspective on this rather general and gloomy picture, supporters were asked at all three interviews how frequently the patient was in certain positive and negative moods ('often', 'sometimes' or 'never'). Changes in the proportion of patients who were reported often to behave in these different ways are shown in Table 55, for those supporters who were seen at each phase of the study. Clearly the trend is for 'positive' moods to become less frequent, particularly being cheerful, alert and interested, with the main changes established by 9 months after the stroke. The proportion of patients exhibiting 'negative' moods even more clearly increased and the situation appeared to worsen with time since the stroke, with the odd exception of reporting aggression. To summarise these changes cumulative scores for positive and negative mood were developed, as explained in the Appendix. Altogether, supporters' views on changes in the patients' moods were unrelated to the severity of the disability as assessed at 1 month after the stroke – a finding in general agreement with research on the relationship between intellectual impairment after stroke and subsequent mood disorder (Warlow *et al.*, 1987). Mood change was not associated with the patient's social class, but there was a tendency for the mood changes of male patients to appear worse

Table 55. *Supporters' reports[a] of the patient's moods before the stroke and at 9 and 18 months after the stroke*

	Before stroke (%)	9 months after (%)	18 months after (%)
Positive moods			
Warm and affectionate	59	51	48
Cheerful	63	45	48
Alert and interested	75	54	45
Appreciative	66	63	62
Negative moods			
Complaining and critical	21	28	37
Aggressive or bad-tempered	13	6	20
Demanding attention	14	25	27
Irritable and easily upset	14	20	32
Depressed	22	25	43

[a] Supporters who were seen at all three interviews ($n = 74$). Figures are the proportion who described the patient as 'often' like this.

than those of female patients – in particular, the rating of male patients' negative moods increased by 2 or more points for 57% of them, compared with 33% of female patients.

Relationship between supporter and patient

Supporters who reported a change in the patient's personality were not more likely to say that their relationship with the patient had changed. In large part this is because the supporters who identified a change in their relationship with the patient (34% of them) were almost equally divided between those who said the relationship had deteriorated and those who felt it was in some way closer or that they cared more. This latter group includes several who were now more 'protective' towards the patient. A son said:

You realise that she is old and one day she will die and that changes it. She is my mother; it [the stroke] brought my attention to it.

And the wife of a man in his sixties felt their relationship had changed:

Perhaps a little because you regard him a little differently. You look at him as someone you have to look after.

None of the wives described their relationship as having become closer, but several took the opposite view:

You can't say you're the same to a person who just sits there and does nothing and can't talk. You can't have the affection you once had when you have to clear up his mess.

Supporters who felt the relationship had deteriorated were not exclusively spouses. And the quality of the relationship before the stroke probably plays a part. A son said, for example, of his mother:

She's always been a burden and a bloody nuisance, but it's worse. I begrudge it more.

Supporters' general descriptions of a change in their relationship with the patient did not capture the extent of change that was found by comparing their responses to specific questions that were asked at each interview. For example, the proportion of supporters who reported that they often looked forward to doing something together with the patient fell from 34% for life before the stroke, to 14% at 18 months after the stroke. The full data are in Table 56, which indicates a more serious decline in the frequency of 'positive' activities, than in the incidence of 'negative' contacts.

As for mood changes, the responses for 'interaction' and 'irritation' have been scored to summary indices of change over time for each patient (see Appendix). The pattern of change in these scores from life before the stroke until 18 months after is presented in Table 57 and shows a rather curious relationship between the severity of disability 1 month after the stroke and changes in the quality of interaction over time. It seems as though the supporters of patients with moderate or severe disability managed to maintain positive interactions as well as did the other supporters, while there was evidence of a decline in 'irritating' contact between these patients and their supporters. Perhaps supporters of patients with severe or moderate disability find daily life more defined and predictable, and find it easier to accept difficulties following stroke, whereas the problems and demands of patients with mild or no disability are less legitimate and more 'irritating'.

No other characteristic of the patient was identified that was consistently related to changes in these scores that reflect the quality of contacts or relationship between the supporter and the patient. Supporters who lived with the patient were not more likely to express either increased negative or positive feelings towards the patient. However, increased irritation was more pronounced among the supporters of older patients (found among 49% of supporters of patients aged 75 or more, but in only 24% of supporters of younger patients). Three-quarters of the supporters of male patients but only half of the supporters of female patients showed declining

Table 56. *Supporters' views[a] on contact with the patient before the stroke and at 9 and 18 months after the stroke*

	Before the stroke (%)	9 months after (%)	18 months after (%)
Positive: 'interaction'			
Had an enjoyable conversation together	80	59	53
Laughed about something together	69	60	54
Felt close to one another	73	60	66
Looked forward to doing something together	34	21	14
Negative: 'irritation'			
Felt cross or angry with the patient	31	30	38
Felt that the patient was interfering too much	10	9	9
Felt tension in relationship with the patient	11	18	22
Had upsetting disagreements with the patient	8	5	9

[a] Supporters who were seen at all three interviews ($n = 74$). Figures are the proportion who reported 'often' having such contacts.

Table 57. *Severity of the patient's disability 1 month after the stroke related to changes in 'interaction' and 'irritation' for supporters*

	Interaction			Irritation		
	Severe/ moderate disability	Mild disability/ normal	All	Severe/ moderate disability	Mild disability/ normal	All
Change in score	(%)	(%)	(%)	(%)	(%)	(%)
+3 or 4	6	5	5	17	15	16
+1 or 2	6	23	15	14	28	22
No change	26	16	20	26	39	33
−1 or 2	48	28	38	29	13	20
−3 or 4	14	28	22	14	5	9
No. of patients (= 100%)	35	39	74	35	39	74

interaction with their patients; and, related to this, 76% of wives of patients had declining scores for interaction compared with 51% of other relatives. Altogether it appears that for the supporters of male patients the experience of companionship and intimacy was more at risk than for supporters of female patients.

The supporters' general rating of the quality of their relationship with the patient declined over time. They were asked to describe their relationship with the patient as 'very happy', 'fairly happy' or 'not happy'. At 1 month after the stroke 64% of supporters described their relationship with the patient before the stroke as very happy; 18 months later only 38% described the relationship as very happy and the proportion who said their relationship was not happy was 15% when it had been 5% for life before the stroke.

Altogether 38% of supporters rated their relationship with the patient in a lower category 18 months after the stroke than they had done for life before the stroke. This proportion was quite constant for patients with different severities of disability at both 1 and 18 months, and was not related to the presence of speech problems. However, only 22% of male supporters but 46% of female supporters rated their relationship as being of a lower quality 18 months after stroke. This appears to be because their relationship with male patients had deteriorated: although the figures are not statistically significant, 52% of the supporters of male patients rated their relationship in a lower category of 'happiness' than they had before the stroke while only 30% of the supporters of women patients did this. Again, these results are affected by the attitudes of the wives of patients, 56% of whom rated their relationship in a lower category. And it appears that the marital relationship is especially prone to deteriorate since, in general, there was no significantly higher rate of deterioration in the relationship of other supporters who lived with the patient.

When the analysis moves from changes in statements about the quality of relationships to comparison of the supporters' relationships with the patients at 18 months after the stroke, the same factors appear to be important; these are shown in Table 58. The supporters' views on their relationship were not associated with the patient's age or social class, but fewer supporters of male patients were 'very happy'. Only 3 men were supporting male patients but among women supporters 43% of those supporting another woman described the relationship as very happy compared with 18% of those who were supporting a man. There was no difference between male and female supporters of women patients in the proportion describing the relationship as very happy. Men who lived with the patient did not differ from other men in their assessments of their

Table 58. *Supporters' views on their relationship with the patient 18 months after the stroke*

	Proportion describing the relationship as 'very happy'	
Sex of supporter:		
Male	57%	(23)[a]
Female	29%	(51)
Sex of patient:		
Male	20%	(30)
Female	50%	(44)
Supporter lives with patient:		
Yes	24%	(32)
No	47%	(42)
Patient's disability at 18 months:		
Moderate/severe	27%	(26)
Mild/normal	43%	(47)

[a] The figures in brackets are the numbers upon which the percentages are based.

relationship with the patient, but only 9% of women who lived with the patient described the relationship as very happy compared with 50% of women supporting patients who lived in their own homes. Eighteen months after the stroke 59% of patients described their relationship with their spouse as very happy and 41% said it was fairly happy – proportions which present a far rosier perspective on the marriage than the spouses, particularly the wives, had. Among the supporters who were married to the patient 30% described their relationship as very happy, 55% as fairly happy and 15% as not very happy. Only 16% of wives described the relationship with the patient as very happy compared with 33% of sisters and 44% of daughters.

Eighteen months after the stroke 42% of patients identified problems caused for their family or friends by the stroke: 20% identified problems for their spouse (that is half of the patients who were living with a spouse), 14% for their children and 10% for siblings, friends or other people. Many felt the illness had caused worry for family or friends, but the specific problems of working to support the patient were usually viewed as a problem, particularly for wives and for daughters.

Among men who identified a problem for their wife, it was reported as:

She's had to work harder. She hasn't been well herself lately, but she carries on. She waits up for an hour after she puts me to bed.

We argue a lot more now. I keep her awake with my chest trouble.

Me! It's sent her up the wall. She's had to spend much more time attending to me and getting things outside.

Well, looking after my wants, my needs, helping me dressing in the morning, doing the shopping on her own and every other bit of business that has to be done, she has to do.

However, only three men felt that their relationship with their wife had been affected by the stroke.

Only three women patients felt that the stroke had caused problems for their spouse and none of these felt their relationship had been affected.

Altogether, 81% of patients felt that their relationship with their children was very happy, 14% that it was fairly happy and 5% judged that it was not very happy. These proportions had not changed in comparison with the patients' assessments at the first interview. When one of the children was the parent's main supporter they viewed their relationship with the patient less happily than the patient did, but not to the same extent as wives diverged from their husbands' (the patients') views. Just over half (52%) of the sons and daughters described their relationship with the patient as very happy, 32% as fairly happy and 16% as not very happy.

The severity of the patient's disability was not a very important influence on the supporter's view of their relationship with the patient. The only significant difference was between supporters of patients with no disability, 59% of whom described the relationship as very happy, and the supporters of all patients with some disability, 30% of whom described their relationship in this way.

The family life of patients with communication problems

Patients with communication problems and their families appear to constitute a particularly disadvantaged group; and the group is larger than that identified in the formal assessments. For example, 18 months after the stroke 32% of patients were recorded as having problems with speech, but 42% of patients themselves described a problem finding words and 48% of supporters said that the patient had difficulty speaking what he or she wanted to say. These discrepancies were also found for a series of patients in Bristol (Wade *et al.*, 1986*a*) and might be due to a variety of conditions including perceptions of disturbed thinking rather than speech problems, or differences in performance when the patient is

Table 59. *Supporters' assessments of difficulties patient had with communication*

	Proportion of supporters who felt the patient had difficulty	
Patient had difficulty:	9 months after stroke	18 months after stroke
Hearing a normal conversation	33% (94)[a]	36% (75)
Understanding a normal conversation	28% (92)	35% (75)
Speaking what he/she wants to say	47% (95)	48% (75)
Reading	39% (95)	47% (70)
Writing	68% (95)	69% (75)
Remembering things	N/A[b]	50% (76)

[a] Figures in brackets are the numbers on which the percentages are based.
[b] N/A, not asked.

tired, or other mild forms of speech disturbance. However, the views of patients and supporters refer to difficulties in speech of whatever cause and are some indication of the frequency of difficulty with communication. The wide range of problems in communication and their persistence over time are indicated in Table 59, which presents the perspective of the patient's supporter.

The views of patients with a speech problem at the third interview, and of their supporters, have been compared with those of the rest to consider any differences in the outcome of the stroke. One-third of patients still had some degree of speech impairment 18 months after the stroke. Not surprisingly, the supporters of speech-impaired patients were more likely to report that the patient conversed much less than before the stroke: 50% of them said this compared with 15% of other supporters. The other main differences in the lives of speech-impaired patients and their families cluster chiefly around the impact on social and family relationships. Some differences are shown in Table 60.

Patients with a speech problem at the third interview were less likely to report that their close family relationships were very happy, although the number of married patients was too small for the difference to be statistically significant. The supporters of speech-impaired patients were generally more likely to feel that their relationship had changed since the stroke. The supporters of men who were speech-impaired were particularly likely to describe their relationship as not very happy: 36% of them did, compared with only 6% of the supporters of male patients who did not have a speech problem.

Table 60. *Some differences between speech-impaired patients and others at 18 months after the stroke*

	Expression at third interview			
Views of patients and supporters	Speech problem		No speech problem	
Patients				
Relationship with spouse is very happy	38%	(8)[a,b]	67%	(21)
Relationship with children is very happy	44%	(16)	94%	(47)
Doing things socially is 'a great problem'	31%	(16)	7%	(61)
Other people treat me differently since the stroke	40%	(15)	13%	(56)
Supporters				
Relationship with the patient has changed	55%	(22)	24%	(51)
Patient shows less interest in family and friends	68%	(22)	38%	(52)

[a]Figures in brackets are the numbers upon which percentages are based.
[b]Not statistically significant.

Speech-impaired patients are overrepresented among patients who make less physical recovery from the stroke (their disability score at 18 months after the stroke was, on average, 5.1 points lower than before the stroke, compared with a mean fall of 2.6 points among other patients). When last seen, 30% of speech-impaired patients were (on Barthel ratings) very severely or severely disabled, compared with 11% of other patients – a difference that has also been found in the Bristol study (Wade *et al.*, 1986a). However, it appears to be the quality of relationships, rather than activities, emotional distress, attitudes to recovery or burden on the supporters, which is most affected by a speech problem. There were no major differences between patients with speech problems and other patients, or between these patients, their supporters and other supporters, over satisfaction with recovery or with life in general. Paradoxically patients with speech problems were more likely than other patients to increase their social activities following stroke: 38% of them did compared with 15% of other patients. This increase was largely because a third of the speech-impaired patients began to attend a social or stroke club regularly; and because half of those who had visitors less than once a week before the stroke were receiving visitors at least weekly 18 months later. However, 53% of patients with a speech problem said they had 'lost interest in things' since the stroke, compared with 26% of other patients; also, as Table 60 shows, patients with a speech problem were more likely to feel that doing things socially, with other people, was a great problem, and to feel that other people had treated them differently since the stroke. Sixty per cent of patients with speech problems said that they felt lonely (compared with 25% of other patients) and 27% reported that there was nobody they felt close to (compared with only 7% of other patients). Altogether, patients who had problems expressing themselves felt more socially isolated, with an average score on this index of 2.0 compared with 1.0 for patients with no speech problem.

There was no indication that supporters of speech-impaired patients were more likely to report changes or restrictions in their work, social or leisure activities; but it appeared that the positive elements of their relationship with the patient had diminished. The interaction scores from before the stroke to 18 months afterwards fell on average by 1.7 points for the supporters of speech-impaired patients but by only 0.6 points for the supporters of other patients.

Helping patients with communication could be intensely frustrating for the supporters. A woman who described her husband as having problems with hearing, speaking and reading said:

It's a severe mental strain. I feel I have to think for him as well as myself.

And the husband of a woman with similar problems exclaimed:

I haven't got much patience; I get irritated with her.

Aspects of the stress on supporters, such as feelings of burden and emotional distress, were in the same direction, suggesting greater stress for the supporters of patients with speech problems. However, this study, like that of Wade and colleagues (1986a), fails to confirm statistically the earlier research of Kinsella and Duffy (1979) in respect of more psychiatric disorder among supporters of speech-impaired patients. It does, though, reiterate the main finding of the earlier research that the effects on supporters are seen particularly in the quality of their relationship with the patient.

It is this experience of deterioration in family and social relationships which principally distinguishes life after stroke for speech-impaired patients and their supporters. Neither group appears well prepared for dealing with the impact of loss of communication on their social relationships. In their support for patients with loss of speech, therapists have an opportunity to help patients and supporters to maintain interest and involvement in family life. This may require the development of new skills or techniques by therapists (e.g. Mulhall, 1978), but such considerations appear to be as important as increasing the sophistication of language assessment and treatment.

Effects on the social and personal life of supporters

The extent to which supporters felt the stroke had changed their family, social and financial lives is shown in Table 61, with reference to the supporter's relationship to the patient.

The supporters' social life

The supporters' social activities scores, as assessed in this study, declined from before the stroke to 18 months later for 60% of supporters. The key factor appears to be whether the supporter lived with the patient, in which case 77% of scores declined compared with 50% when the patient and supporter lived in their own households. The extent of the decline was not associated with the supporter's sex or relationship to the patient, nor significantly with the severity of the patient's initial disability – although only 9% of the supporters of patients with no disability reduced their activities by 3 or more points compared with 38% of the supporters of patients with more severe disability.

There was some increase and decrease in all activities, but going out to see family and friends exhibited the only significant decline in frequency, as shown in Table 62.

Although the social activities scores of the wives of patients did not decline significantly further than those of other supporters, wives were in all respects more likely to feel that their social lives had changed since the stroke, as shown in Table 61. Some wives described the change in their social activities as 'complete' and were distressed by this. For example, a woman, whose husband had moderate disability had had to give up her social club and said:

I resented it because it was the only thing I had.

And the wife of a man with mild disability said:

I feel I'm getting an awful bore. I can't get out and do anything.

However, other wives and many other supporters appeared to accept the limitations with equanimity, with remarks like:

I've got the telephone and that makes a lot of difference.

I can't go anywhere and leave Fred for any length of time. [How do you feel about that?] It's not worried me much really.

I just take it as it comes. I've got no intent to go out and leave her.

Table 61. *Relationship of supporter to patient and effects of the stroke on their lives*

	Proportion of supporters describing life as affected by the stroke				
Aspect of life affected	Wife (%)	Husband (%)	Daughter (%)	Son (%)	All supporters (%)
Social life	63	43	42	31	42
Leisure activities	58	43	37	31	36
Social activities 'severely' restricted	47	14	16	8	21
Relationship with other family or friends	16	14	26	38	21
Caused problems for other members of family	40	14	26	31	27
Financial circumstances	32	29	37	15	26
No. of supporters (= 100%)	20	7	19	13	75

Table 62. *Changes in the frequency with which supporters went to visit family or friends*

Frequency of visits in the 3 months before the interview	Before stroke (%)	9 months after (%)	18 months after (%)
Never	12	13	23
1–2 times	4	15	13
3–12 times	14	26	26
Weekly or more	70	46	38
No. of supporters (= 100%)	73	74	74

Well, I've never given it much thought. We didn't go out much anyway.

Altogether, 21% of supporters described their social lives as 'severely' restricted by the stroke, 7% as 'fairly' restricted, 26% as 'a little' restricted, and 46% as 'not at all' restricted. The wives of patients were more likely to view their lives as severely restricted, as Table 61 showed. In general, 41% of supporters who lived with the patient viewed their lives as severely restricted compared with only 6% of the supporters of patients who lived in their own homes. But among supporters who lived with the patient, 50% of women felt their social life was severely restricted compared with 20% of men. Although this difference was not statistically significant, it reflects a fairly consistent difference in the experience of stroke. The severity of the patient's disability at 1 month and 18 months after the stroke was not clearly related to the perception of social restrictions.

The supporters' other relationships

Only 27% of supporters said that the stroke had caused problems for other members of the family. Of these supporters, 65% described problems for a daughter or a son, 20% for a brother or sister and only 10% for their spouse. For their children, a major concern was the extra work they did, but there were also concerns about the extra worry it caused them and about restrictions on their lives. For example, the husband of one patient depended upon support from his daughter, who lived at home, since he went out to work. He felt that his daughter:

Normally she would have been at work; she would have had more social life.

Similarly, other supporters with jobs or other commitments relied upon help from others. A man who lived with his father and two sisters made the point:

Because I am at work a lot of the demands in the day are made on them [his sisters].

And a similar point was made by a harassed, self-employed man about the support his wife gave to his mother:

She's had to live with me, go and see Mum. She's had a lot more work to do dealing with Mum's stuff.

Although these supporters have pointed out consequences for other members of the family, the proportion of other family members adversely affected by the stroke seems quite low, and it underscores the point that the responsibility for providing help and support appears to fall mostly on a single individual. The failure of others to share the caring with the supporter was noted in Chapter 6, when supporters commented on the help that they felt family and friends could have given. This lack of shared support appears to be a major reason for the stroke affecting the supporter's relationship with other family members and friends.

Altogether only 21% of supporters felt that their relationship with anyone else had changed since the stroke, and siblings were the largest group. Only 3 supporters felt the stroke had caused a serious strain on their marriage, and 3 that they now saw less of their friends because of the stroke. The sister of a patient in an unsatisfactory nursing home reported that she and her husband:

We've had words. We can't sit down and talk about it without getting heated.

And a woman who supported her mother at home until a place was found in sheltered housing felt that her mother:

... more or less took over my friends. I haven't really got any close friends now. They got that they didn't come – she used to be nasty towards them. She did make a bit of nuisance of herself with the neighbours and with my friends.

So, supporters felt that some of their relationships had changed because others were too little involved with the patient, and some felt that they had changed because others were too involved. Altogether, when the patient was not their spouse 67% of supporters described their marriage as very happy, 27% as fairly happy and only 6% as not happy 18 months after the stroke. In this respect there was no significant difference between the marriages of daughters and sons of the patient. Similarly, most supporters (87%) described relationships with their children as very happy; but the daughters of stroke patients seemed to have more problems – only 69% described their relationship with their children as very happy compared with 94% of other supporters.

Work and money

Among the supporters 18 months after the stroke, 4 had given up work and 6 had changed their job in some way since the stroke. The numbers are small and the difference is not statistically significant, but, amongst those who were employed at the time of the stroke, some change had been experienced by 42% of the daughters of stroke patients but by only 20% of other supporters. Only one person who, before the stroke, worked full-time had given up work. However, 5 of the 6 people who had made changes in their job had been working 30 or more hours a week before the stroke. The daughter of a woman who lived alone:

... had to cut my hours down at work so I could see her every day. I work half day now. [Interviewer: How do you feel about that?] It's one of them things; it's just got to be.

The wife of one patient had her own art studio; she said:

I've given up my drawing school. But I've started a children's class here now. [Interviewer: How do you feel about that?] I don't resent it completely but obviously you're sorry.

Other supporters gave up or changed work temporarily following the stroke; 18% of those who were employed did this in the month after the stroke. This was difficult for some because their employment was inflexible, and a problem for others because they lost work and income. Altogether 26% of supporters said that their finances were affected by the stroke. These supporters included those who had changed their jobs, as the daughter of one woman patient illustrates:

I was on unpaid leave after the stroke. I could not claim sick pay or anything like that. That worried her [patient] too; the fact that I was off work and not earning.

However, there were a series of new expenses that supporters, particularly those living with the patient (34% of whom said the illness had affected their finances) had to face:

Because we're having to pay a gardener. Also we used to do all our own decorating, now we have to pay the builder to do all the jobs around the house. We bought chairs, to make him feel no different – the same as the hospital chair, but in the same material as our furniture.

Supporters identified other new expenses such as travel costs for more frequent visits, new clothes because the patients had changed weight, and particularly costs associated with extra heating. Altogether, the financial consequences of the stroke were felt fairly equally by those with different relationships to the patient, by male and female supporters, all social classes, and across the range of severities of disability.

The single help with financial difficulties that was mentioned by some carers was the attendance allowance. The wife of a patient with severe disability said:

I find that I get paid the night and day allowance but you spend it; all sorts of things you have to spend the money on – washing powder, disinfectant.

And the wife of another patient noted:

We get the attendance allowance so I would say we were just about the same really. You don't spend so much on pleasures but more on heating, 'phone bills and so on.

Altogether, 24% of patients said they received an attendance allowance, and this proportion increased with increasing severity of the stroke from 22% of those with mild disability, to 38% of those with moderate and 63% of patients with severe disability. No one who lived alone received this help, but 57% of patients who lived with their spouse did. Seventeen per cent of patients who received the attendance allowance said they were still bothered with money worries, as did 21% of other patients, some of whom were frustrated applicants for allowances. A 69-year-old man with moderate disability spent most of one year shuffling between applications for exemption from vehicle excise duty, mobility allowance and attendance allowance – all to no avail. He concluded that by the next time vehicle excise duty was due:

I shall have disposed of the vehicle, requested the doctor to visit me as I cannot walk, applied for Meals on Wheels, and resigned myself to the life of a hermit, confined to four walls and a garden. Courtesy of the DHSS. I think their booklet 'Help for Handicapped People' should have received the Booker Prize. It is the best piece of fiction I've read for a long time.

The proportion of patients with money worries was not associated with the patient's age, sex, social class or the severity of the disability.

SUMMARY

This chapter looked at aspects of change in the everyday life of patients and their supporters – at home, at work and in leisure, among family and friends, and particularly the relationship between the patient and the supporter.

Home and social activities   Nearly everyone settles into a pattern of doing less housework after stroke – 80% of patients were doing less and, although change was not associated with sex or age, men, older patients and those living with others were doing less housework than other patients 18 months after stroke. Relatively few patients, and mostly women, regarded housework as a problem. Levels of both housework and social activities were broadly related to the patient's disability. Overall, there was little change in social activities, mainly because levels of family contact were maintained. However, patients aged under 75 had reduced their activities more than older patients, in part because people who were doing more before the stroke subsequently gave up more activities. The supporters tended to view changes in the patient's social activities as more dramatically in decline. Although it appeared that patients who had been emotionally distressed after the stroke were no more or less likely to reduce social activities, the supporters' statements clearly indicated a greater reduction in social participation among patients who had been rated as emotionally distressed 1 month after the stroke. Most patients did not regard their social life 18 months after stroke as a serious problem, largely because many had little interest in social involvement outside their family. However, among patients who felt that mixing socially was a problem, this was almost always attributed to some consequence of the stroke.

Personal distress Levels of emotional distress among patients tended to remain fairly constant over the course of the study; 18 months after the stroke one-third of patients said they woke up feeling depressed. Patients with moderate or severe disability were more emotionally distressed, but disability was not related to feelings of social isolation or to change in these scores. There appeared to be a high risk of social isolation after the stroke, particularly felt by certain groups; three-fifths of the middle-class patients described themselves as feeling lonely compared with a quarter of the patients classified as working-class. Although the research identified a low level of feelings of stigma among patients, it appeared again that more middle-class patients felt they were treated as inferior. At 18 months 45% of the patients felt they had changed as a person since the stroke but 62% of the supporters thought this. Supporters recorded a marked increase in negative moods (being miserable, irritable and depressed) among patients.

Relationship between supporter and patient Over the period following the stroke there was a clear fall in the frequency with which supporters reported 'positive' activities with the patient. Changes in the quality of 'interaction', and in the relationship between supporter and patient, were not related to the severity of the patient's disability following the stroke but appeared to deteriorate, particularly if the supporter was the patient's wife. 'Irritating' contacts, unexpectedly, were somewhat less likely to increase among supporters of patients with moderate or severe disability. Supporters who were married to the patient, and especially wives, had much less happy views of their relationship than did the patients; on the other hand, few of the patients felt their marital relationship had been affected by the stroke.

Patients with communication problems A high proportion of patients saw themselves, and were viewed by their supporters, as having residual problems with communication. These patients and their families were afflicted not only with these problems, but speech-impaired patients were also more disabled than others. However, it was particularly in the quality of their relationships and in feelings of social isolation that speech-impaired patients were disadvantaged. For supporters there was a marked decline in the quality of their interaction with the patient, and there were indications of greater stress among the supporters of patients with speech problems.

Social life and relationships of supporters   A majority of supporters, particularly those living with the patient, reduced their social activities following the stroke; this was most marked for going out to visit family and friends. A fifth of supporters described their life as severely restricted by the stroke. Again wives were especially likely to feel this, but, more generally, 41% of people who lived with the patient reported that their social activities had been severely restricted compared with only 6% of the supporters of patients who lived in their own home. Supporters were concerned about the effects of the stroke on other family members who cared for or about the patient, but in most cases they did not feel that the stroke had significantly damaged other relationships.

Money   More than a quarter of the supporters who had been working before the stroke had given up or changed their job in some way since the stroke, although only one person had given up full-time work. Altogether, a quarter of the supporters reported that they had suffered a financial loss since the stroke, in some cases because of a loss of income but also because of new expenses for travel, clothes, heating, etc. Among patients, 1 in 4 received an attendance allowance; this proportion rose with increasing severity of the stroke, and covered more than half the married patients. Nevertheless, a fifth of patients said they had money worries.

Many of the results in this chapter show that for both patients and supporters the physical disability caused by stroke is generally a limiting condition, but not one that dictates response to the stroke or the psychosocial consequences. In particular, the lives of supporters seem to be influenced greatly by the nature and quality of their relationship with the patient. The attitudes of supporters and the main influences on coping with the stroke are the focus for the next chapter.

CHAPTER EIGHT

Caring and coping with stroke

The burden of caring and the stress on carers has in recent years moved to centre stage in debates – scholarly, popular and political – about the conditions for care in the community of people with chronic physical and mental disability. There is concern about the health of carers, about the financial, social and emotional impoverishment caused by caring, and about the handicapping of carers', principally women's, lives (Anderson, 1987). Among the cultural expectations associated with caring, a persistent theme seems to be that caring is essentially women's work (Finch and Groves, 1983). Whatever the implications of this expectation, it is evident that the job of caring for a disabled person is surrounded by cultural assumptions: about who should care; about mutual and family obligations; and, particularly when caring is predominantly for older people, about its value and importance for society.

Caring may be taken on as a 'natural' response to loving someone, as a duty or obligation, or out of guilt and a lack of alternatives. These attitudes to caring will influence responses to the patient's needs and to caring tasks; and they present complex factors mediating between caring and how supporters feel about this. This chapter begins with a preliminary discussion of attitudes to caring, followed by an analysis of the supporters' experience of burden. It continues by looking at the role of information in helping patients and supporters to cope, and concludes with the views of patients and supporters on the outcome 18 months after stroke.

Attitudes to caring

At 1 month after the stroke the common view among supporters was that they would be the principal source of help and care. The wife of one 60-year-old man said:

I don't know how well he's going to be before they let him home, but whatever help he wants he'll get from me.

Another wife identified herself and the main jobs she thought would be important:

My help – we manage quite well. Getting him dressed, washed, cooking and washing.

These practical tasks, mainly housework, were the sort of help that most supporters thought the patients would need. District nurses, together with home helps and Meals on Wheels, were the services that supporters most commonly expected to provide other support. A small number of supporters mentioned their concern, however, that the patient would not accept help from these statutory services. The son of one stoical First World War veteran said:

He won't have a home help or Meals on Wheels. I've asked him to have a home help; that would take some of the weight off me. I can only provide so much, I'm nearly an Old Age Pensioner myself. What about my welfare?

Several other supporters mentioned at this stage that they would take on or carry on caring but, for various reasons, were worried about the effects on their own health. Some regarded themselves as the only available choice as carer; either there was no one else or it was not acceptable to disrupt the lives of others – particularly children. One patient had a wife who worked in a residential home; she gave an accurate prediction of the year ahead:

I will have to give up my job. I've asked for a home help; I'll stay home and look after him. I've got a daughter but I won't ask her to do too much because she's got two young children and a husband.

Another wife commented:

There'll only be me here. My daughter has to go to work. She might help at the weekend. I think he [patient] would be embarrassed if my daughter had to help. Her heart would be in it, but I wouldn't like to have to rely on her for that. That's my biggest problem: how will we cope? I don't like to ask my family because they're all younger with young children to look after.

In response to a specific question at the first interview 70% of the supporters said that they had some worries about helping the patient following the stroke. This proportion was not clearly related to severity of the patient's disability. Other characteristics of the patient – age, sex, social class – did not appear to affect the proportion of supporters with worries, nor were these relevant characteristics of the supporters. Supporters who lived with the patient were not more likely to specify worries, but the supporter's view on the quality of his or her relationship with the patient before the stroke was important: 88% of those who described this relationship as 'fairly happy' or 'not very happy' identified specific worries, compared with 63% of supporters who described their relationship with the patient before the stroke as 'very happy'. The significance of their relationship with the patient before the stroke probably lies in its importance to supporters compared with their other relationships. Perhaps there is a keener sense of the limits to which they are prepared to give help. The son of a woman whose communication was seriously impaired had a wife who was ill; about helping his mother, he said:

There's got to be conditions on that about the wife's health; if she is ill I'm not going to rush up here. Some officialdom might imagine in their wildest dreams that they can ship her [patient] off to us, but it's just not feasible – under all circumstances my wife comes first.

In various guises, the demands made by the patient on the supporter's time and, therefore, ability to fulfil other commitments, appeared to be one of the major worries for supporters. In part, supporters were worried that caring for the patient would disrupt the lives of other family. A daughter put the problem succinctly:

That I will not be able to cope with the situation when she gets home. It's really the conflict I feel between providing adequate help for my mother and having extra stress on myself and my own family.

This conflict between the needs of the patient and the commitments of the supporter caused several supporters to worry that the care they provided for the patient was not adequate. The sister of one patient and the daughter of another were caught between the need to work and the uncomfortable thought that without them the patient might need to go into residential care.

I'm out at work all day so I couldn't have her living here. I enjoy my work and need the money. I wouldn't like to be at home all day. We'll do all we can to help her. I don't want her living with me on a permanent basis. I don't think it would work. She's been good to us. I wouldn't let her go into a home.

Just him being on his own ... I couldn't give up my job to look after him, I'd go round the bend; but I'd never leave him on his own. I just wish he had someone else that could share the burden with me. I'm the only one left. I wish I knew he was being looked after and that; I'd hate him to go into a home.

Most of the worries about caring were about effects on the patient and other family members; they were also about the effects on the supporter's health. When supporters mentioned worries about the strain of caring or about effects on their health, it tended to refer to a concern about being able to help the patient. The wife of a patient who was both severely disabled and without speech said her main worry was:

That I'm going to have enough strength to cope with it. I'm hoping I'm going to keep in good health because if you haven't got that you haven't got anything. I just pray that my mind doesn't go. This happens when you been amongst strokes and that kind of thing.

Altogether, the supporters' assessment of their health before the stroke was not associated with the proportion of them who mentioned worries about helping the patient. Possibly, this is because there are simply so many potential difficulties for carers, only some of which make physical demands on them. One supporter put her worries about helping into the frame of her worries about the patient:

I'm worried about her financially. I'm worried about whether she's going to be able to cope physically and look after the dog. How far she's going to become depressed about the further limitations on her life. I'm worried about the possi-bility of a further stroke that might disable her more. I'm as worried as I can be about every part of her life. I think it is going to be extremely difficult but I try not to let her see I'm worried because she is worried enough herself about how she's going to manage.

Coping with caring

Eighteen months after the stroke two-thirds of patients were less indepen-dent in activities of daily living than they had been before the stroke. Their supporters were asked at the third interview about the help they were then giving the patients. In comparison with life before the stroke nearly half (45%) said they were now spending 'much more' time helping with practical jobs such as getting the patient about, bathing, shopping and doing housework; 21% of supporters said they were spending 'slightly more' time on this, 25% said there had been no change and 9% that they were giving less practical help than they had before the stroke. It was clear that spouses and the few other supporters who lived with the patient were more likely to report spending much more time giving the patient practical help – 64% of them said this compared with only 35% of the supporters of patients who were living in their own homes.

It is possible that giving routine practical help becomes established soon after the patient comes home from hospital and then fails to change with the patient's condition. Reported changes in help given were associ-ated with the patient's Barthel score 1 month after stroke (57% of the supporters of patients with severe or moderate disability reported giving much more help 18 months after the stroke compared with 33% of the supporters of patients who had mild or no disability), but were not related to the Barthel score at 18 months after the stroke.

Male and female patients appeared to cause the supporter to make similar increases in the level of their practical help, while characteristics of the supporters, such as age, sex and social class, were not related to their assessments of how much more practical help they were giving. However, there was a major difference between male and female supporters in their views about whether any increase in helping caused particular problems or difficulties; only 44% of men said the increased help had caused problems compared with 79% of women. This was not because women were caring for more disabled patients – they were not; nor was it simply because more of the women were caring for men – sex of the patient made no difference to the proportion with problems. Perhaps women were doing more than men, and doing it more frequently, or perhaps they were stretched by other commitments to home, work and family. But perhaps also they are more inclined to identify and respond to problems (see Pearlin and Schooler, 1978), particularly emotional and social difficulties.

Altogether, two-thirds of the supporters who had increased their practical help said it caused them some difficulty. This was not associated with the supporter's age or social class nor with those characteristics of the patient; nor, perhaps surprisingly, with the patient's disability scores at either 1 or 18 months following the stroke. The nature of these difficulties gives some clue to this apparent discrepancy between disability and the problem caused by helping more.

Only two of the supporters made direct reference to difficulties caused by lifting or the sheer physical capacity required to do things for the patient. However, the single most common problem was the related one of tiredness, which was mentioned by about a quarter of the supporters, all of them women. Two of the wives associated the problem with being older themselves:

I get tired, which is only natural because I'm coming up to 68. It isn't as though you're young is it? I'm nowhere near methodical like I used to be because you haven't got the time to be like it.

Just that I'm getting older and I'm getting very weary. It does put a lot of strain on the wife, doesn't it?

The constant, repetitive nature of 'strain' was referred to by several other supporters. Among those who did not live with the patient, several mentioned the problem of finding time, as well as energy, to visit and meet the patient's needs. The resources of one daughter were stretched by the problems of getting to her mother's flat in Thamesmead:

I'm there practically every afternoon. I'd much rather be at home. You come out of work absolutely exhausted and all you want to do is get home. It's three bus rides from here to Thamesmead.

The problem of being tied, of being available at certain times, rather than the tasks involved, were sources of difficulty for other supporters. A woman caring for her severely disabled husband identified the main difficulties as:

I don't get the sleep that you should have. When you're stuck in for so long you get short-tempered. You just can't put your coat on and run up the shops.

Other difficulties mentioned by the supporters included being 'on call' all the time, feeling worried or depressed about how the patient was coping with practical tasks, and having too little time for other people, principally spouses. Practical tasks were also taken by some supporters to include housekeeping and financial matters. Sorting out finances could be a constant strain, as the son of a patient who had owned her own home found out:

Directly, not much more time, but indirectly seeing to her house and finance, a lot. Dealing with the DHSS, with the [nursing] home, the insurance company, decorators, workmen. Trying to sell the house. Getting bits and pieces to the home. Calming her [mother] down, calming the home down, calming me down. Stopping my wife from murdering her. Telling my brother to get stuffed. Dealing with welfare people, hospitals and doctors.

Compared with all this perhaps pushing the wheelchair, washing clothes and helping the patient to dress are seen as lesser problems; or, if they are difficult for the supporter, then nursing and social services or a neighbour step in to help.

At both the second and third interviews the main approach to identifying the principal source of distress among supporters was to ask them: 'Of all the things we have discussed what difficulty or problem has upset you most?' Their responses have been coded into the general categories seen in Table 63.

The direct, practical and physical problems of caring are the main cause of upset for only 1 in 6 supporters. In response to a specific question at the second interview at 9 months after the stroke, none of the supporters said these practical jobs caused a 'great problem'. It was more distressing for supporters to see the patient dependent and restricted; and this helplessness among some patients appeared particularly striking to supporters at

Table 63. *Reports from supporters about the difficulty or problem that upset them most*

	After 9 months (%)	After 18 months (%)
Nothing/not distressed (now)	16	15
Social restrictions on supporter (inc. loss of companionship with patient)	15	14
Isolation of supporter (esp. lack of support from family/services)	8	7
Patient's mood/personality	19	7
Patient's (physical) dependency, helplessness, lack of recovery	15	30
Practical problem for supporter:		
General	6 ⎫	4 ⎫
Dealing with incontinence	2 ⎪	2 ⎪
Communicating with patient	2 ⎬ 17	8 ⎬ 15
Lifting	2 ⎪	1 ⎪
Doing housework	5 ⎭	0 ⎭
Patient's housing/accommodation	5	5
Other problems of patient	3	3
Other problems of supporter	2	4
No. of supporters (= 100%)	87	73

the third interview, possibly because by then few expected the further improvement that they had been hoping for 9 months earlier. For the supporter, this was how the patient was going to be; and, as the wife of a man in his seventies said, she was most upset:

Seeing him like this [moderately disabled]. Sometimes I think it would be better if he had been taken when he had the stroke. It's no life at all for him, and it could go on for years like this.

It was, not surprisingly, difficult for some supporters to accept that the active partnership of many years was over. One couple had continued working in their early seventies, but now the woman was only able to get about in her wheelchair. Her husband was upset most:

To see the helplessness of a woman that's always been so active. She was able and so capable. She was never no trouble to me physically.

Inevitably, many of the supporters who lived with patients who were unable to walk were doing much more practical work, but the poignancy or distress for them was clearly generated by the patient's predicament:

To think that he can't walk. He lived in the garden; if he could walk that would be the best thing. Sometimes he looks out the window and you know what he's thinking.

Supporters, then, often felt sorry for patients who were often distressed themselves. The daughter of a woman who was rated as having no disability was upset by:

How much it depresses her. To see her in these depressive states, that upsets me. And I don't like her feeling incapable.

However, the supporter's distress at the patient's distress was not always so benign. It appeared, in particular at the second interview, that the patient's mood or change in personality was a source of both stress and upset to the main supporter. For example, the two spouses quoted above who were upset by seeing the patient's loss of independence had different concerns at 9 months after the stroke:

This change of character; but everybody has said that this is something that is so common with this complaint.

He goes at me. There's not a day goes by he doesn't go at me. Every day I go to the hospital I think 'What am I going to be greeted with this time?

This woman was one among several supporters (though she did not know this) who were feeling tired and upset by the patient's bad humour:

When she can't see right from wrong; she drives me mad at times.

I don't really know. I can't express it – very difficult . . . cussedness I suppose really. He can be very cussed at times – this is when he does cause me stress – when he's awkward.

The wife of a patient who was both moderately disabled and had a major loss of speech expressed a sentiment shared by many of the married couples that the stroke had disrupted their plans for the future together and this was somehow not fair:

To feel that Jack's like this. I get upset to think we've worked hard together to enjoy this time of life and now this has happened. You feel there's no justice sometimes.

Among the different ways in which the stroke affected the lives of supporters, the restrictions of their social life and free use of time were the most upsetting, being mentioned by 1 in 6 of the supporters at both the second and third interviews. Occasionally, social activities were lost because they had previously been joint activities with the patient; as a wife said:

I do miss going out together like we used to. I do get a bit depressed over that.

And the husband of a woman who had become housebound said he was most upset because:

There's quite a lot of things that we can't do together, like holidays, going for walks together, all of them little things, where we used to have a rave-up.

More commonly, though, supporters had opportunities for social activity but were not able to use them. Some were unable to pursue previous interests, as one woman reported:

The fact that I can't socialise, go to classes, mix with people. I used to do that when I was at work.

Others were distressed because they felt themselves to be trapped by the stroke, tied to the patient's needs and to the home in which the patient lived. A son described the most distressing aspect of his father's stroke as:

Being tied to the house itself, because that's where he is.

And, echoing the woman who described the illness as unjust, another wife said the main upset was:

Just that you can't get out really. You've come to an age when you could have a bit of enjoyment in life and you can't, you're stopped.

In both of these cases, and in most others, supporters appeared to be tied to the patients by composite bonds of affection and guilt, not because the patient needed constant nursing care. However, the patients may have been dependent on the supporters for social contact and daily tasks such as shopping. Perhaps feelings of guilt were more prevalent among people who did not live with the patient, who had their own lives to lead. Two supporters in this position described what upset them most as:

It's always on your mind, sort of thing. She's always saying she gets lonely. I always feel when I go out, I shouldn't be going because she can't go out.

We never seem to have no time to ourselves. After work we go straight to the hospital. She has taken our pleasure time. If we don't go down there we feel guilty.

This impression that perhaps people who did not live with the patient felt more pressure or guilt to do more appears to be supported in responses to a question posed about 9 months after the stroke. Supporters were asked whether they felt able to do as much as they wanted for the patient, or whether they wished they could do more. Altogether, 44% of supporters said they wished they could do more, but this proportion was only 33% of those who lived with the patient compared with 54% of the supporters not living with the patient. Associated with this, the proportion of people who felt they were doing enough to help the patient increased with the supporter's age, from 35% of those aged less than 45 to 71% of supporters aged 65 and over. Of the spouses 70% felt they were

able to do as much as they wanted for the patient, but only 49% of
children who were supporters said this; however, this difference was not
statistically significant. The proportion of supporters who wished they
could do more was not related to the sex of either patient or supporter or
to the patient's Barthel score.

Supporters wanted to do a variety of things for the patients, from
practical help and improving their social activities, especially by taking
them out more, to wishing they could help with finding the patients more
suitable accommodation. They were prevented from doing more by their
own lack of energy or health, by lack of facilities or support from others,
by the weather and lack of public transport, by practical problems in
getting the patient about, and by their own commitments to work or
family.

The burden of caring

Supporters were reluctant to describe the help they gave as a problem –
the proportion who described the help they gave as causing 'no problem'
was 77% for those helping with housework, 74% among those helping
with self-care tasks and 70% among supporters who helped the patient to
get about. Generally, supporters considered this help to be 'their job'.
Possibly those who found the tasks overwhelming were no longer doing
them 9 months after the stroke. But as Chapter 6 showed, most patients
were receiving care and support primarily from the main supporter. The
'selection hypothesis' is, therefore, unlikely, and it appears that most
supporters accommodate to the practical tasks in caring.

No common thread was found which consistently distinguished the
supporters who found the help they gave caused a problem, from those
who did not. The severity of the patient's disability was related to the
identity of the supporter giving help (see Chapter 6), but, among those
giving help, severity of disability was not generally associated with saying
helping was a problem. The age and sex of the patient were not associated
with the supporter's identification of a problem, nor was whether or not
the supporter lived with the patient. The spouses who helped patients
were consistently more likely than children of the patient to say helping
caused a problem, but none of the differences were statistically significant.
Perhaps spouses both do more caring and suffer more restrictions, but
they are more likely to see this as a natural, expected role that does not
merit defining as a problem. Neither the sex nor social class of supporters
was related to their responses about the degree of problem caused by
helping with practical tasks. However, when these attitudes to help are

Table 64. *Supporters problems with helping the patient and their assessment of burden*

	Proportion who described the 'burden' as moderate or large	
Helping with:	Helping patient causes no problem	Helping patient causes some problem
Getting about	31% (32)[a]	57% (14)
Self-care	29% (34)	67% (12)
Use of the toilet	27% (11)	86% (7)
Communication	27% (41)	70% (10)
Housework	31% (54)	44% (16)

[a] Figures in brackets are the numbers on which percentages are based.

considered in relation to the supporters' more general assessments of the burden caused by caring, it becomes clear that the concept of burden is not subsumed by these categories of practical help.

At the second interview almost one-third of the supporters described the burden caused by the help and support they were giving the patient as 'moderate' or 'large'. This proportion was not significantly associated with finding the help they gave with housework or with getting the patient about to be a problem; but those supporters who had 'some problem' helping with self-care, use of the toilet or with communication were more likely to describe caring as a moderate or large burden. The figures are in Table 64.

Supporters were asked about the burden caused by the help and support they were giving, but these results suggest the need to look further at what supporters understood or meant by the concept of 'burden'. It was clear that their responses were usually framed in terms of the patient as a person, rather than in terms of the work that had to be done. The word 'burden' is linked to negative value judgements, which some supporters were not prepared to apply. The wife of one patient who was moderately disabled and disoriented said that the help and support she gave caused 'no burden':

Not when it's someone you care for.

And another woman who helped a male friend with dressing, feeding and housework responded that this was not a burden because:

I've only got myself. If I didn't do that for him what would I do all day in the flat?

The wife of a patient with severe disability said:

I don't look on it as burden.

And a husband noted:

If you do it for your own wife how can you say it's a burden?

So, referring to help given to the patient as a burden is not legitimate in some relationships.

In cases where the caring *was* felt to cause a burden the effort and exhaustion of the work involved was mentioned by some supporters; but other aspects of caring appeared to be the cause at least as often as tiredness or health problems. Among the main causes of burden were general worry about the patient and financial problems for the supporter. The cost of travelling to the patient's home was a concern. The daughter who took three buses from work to her mother's flat said caring was a large burden:

I find it an awful struggle financially as well as physically.

And a man who came over to Greenwich every weekend from Essex said helping was a moderate burden because:

The cost of petrol and things we bring her – out of one wage. My wife has to go without things.

Restrictions on daily life were the most frequently mentioned causes of burden, particularly restrictions on the time and freedom that supporters had for themselves. Supporters made a variety of comments explaining this:

You always feel that you are on your mettle to be on hand.

The fact that I can't go away for any length of time, when from the point of view of my career I probably should.

You're not free to go and visit family and that sort of thing.

However, some supporters do not view helping as a burden even when their lives are extremely restricted. The daughter of a woman who moved into her home after the stroke said:

She's not really a burden to me. I know I can't go out or anything but I can't say it's a burden.

So, which supporters of which patients did feel that the help and support they gave was a burden? For this analysis the experience of supporters up to the third interview, 18 months after the stroke, has been used. Altogether the supporters' experience of burden increased greatly

Table 65. *Supporters' reports of the burden caused by helping the patient*

Help and support given to the patient caused:	Before stroke (%)	9 months after stroke (%)	18 months after stroke (%)
No burden	74	36	48
A little burden	17	35	15
A moderate burden	5	20	20
A large burden	4	9	17
No. of supporters (= 100%)	75	75	75

following the stroke. This is shown in Table 65, which looks at responses from supporters – seen at the third interview – at different stages following the stroke. There was little change in the general picture between 9 and 18 months after the stroke but the reported burden was greater at the third interview for 23% of supporters, and appeared to have declined between the second and third interviews for 28% of them.

The general picture parallels the pattern of change in functional recovery among patients, arriving after 9 months at a plateau, but perceived burden had relatively little relationship to the patient's disability scores. Patients whose score had fallen by 3 or more points since before the stroke were less likely to be described as 'no burden' (33% were, compared with 57% of the patients with less or no deterioration in their score), but there was no relationship between the extent of change in disability scores and the size of the reported burden.

By 18 months after the stroke there was only a difference between those patients with no disability and the rest in the extent to which their supporters described helping them as a burden: 18% of patients with no disability were receiving help which caused the supporters a moderate or large burden compared with 45% of patients with some measured disability. The mobility, self-care and disability scores of patients whose help caused no or a little burden were not significantly different from those of patients whose support caused a moderate or large burden. Other characteristics of the stroke – side of weakness, first or subsequent stroke, loss of speech – were also not associated with subjective feelings of burden among supporters.

Help given to male patients was no more or less likely to cause a burden, nor was the patient's age or marital status an important factor. However, the help given to working-class patients was described as a large burden by 21% of their supporters compared with only 6% of the supporters of patients classified as middle-class. This difference is not statistically significant but possibly it reflects a difference in the prepared-ness of supporters to label patients as a burden – although the social class of supporters did not relate to their perception of burden. Nor were the supporters of working-class patients different from those of middle-class patients with regard to age, sex or relationship to the patient. This suggests that some characteristic of working-class patients may have been important. It was reported in previous chapters that there were no social class differences in disability scores; but as reported in Chapter 7 more working-class patients had high levels of emotional distress. And one-third of the patients who scored 4 or more for emotional distress had supporters who described the help they gave as causing a large burden, compared with one-tenth of the supporters of patients who scored 3 or less on the measure of emotional distress. The greater distress of working-class patients appears to make a contribution to the supporters' feelings of burden.

The patient's level of emotional distress was consistently reflected in the supporters' assessments of the frequency of negative moods in the patient (see Appendix), the correlation between the two measures being sig-nificant at the 0.01 level ($r = 0.34$). The supporters' assessments of the patient's moods and of the quality of the contact between patient and supporter were strongly related to subjective feelings of burden, as shown in Table 66. Not surprisingly, the table also shows that the supporters' view of their relationship with the patient is less positive when they feel that the caring imposes on them a moderate or large burden. But what is the direction of this relationship? Do feelings of burden cause deterior-ation in the relationship or does the quality of the relationship affect feelings of burden? Data from the first interview suggest the plausibility of the latter explanation: only 25% of those supporters who said their relationship with the patient before the stroke was very happy then said, 18 months later, that the burden of caring was moderate or large, compared with 63% of the supporters who described their relationship before the stroke as fairly happy or not happy. The quality of the previous relationship is not the only important determinant; supporters who rated their health before the stroke as less good were more likely to find helping the patient a moderate or large burden. The proportion who felt this increased from 22% of those who rated their health for their age as excellent to 71% of those who described it as poor.

The demographic characteristics of the supporters appeared to be less important predictors of subjective burden than their health and their relationship with the patient before the stroke. There were no differences

Table 66. *Some determinants and correlates of supporters' perceived burden*

	Supporter feels help and support for the patient has caused:	
	No/little burden	Moderate/large burden
Supporters' ratings		
Before stroke own health was excellent or good for age	66%	41%
Before stroke relationship with patient was 'very happy'	78%	41%
At 18 months relationship with patient is 'very happy'	53%	11%
Average scores at 18 months for		
Interaction	5.9	2.8
Irritation	1.7	3.9
Positive mood	6.2	3.6
Negative mood	3.1	7.0
No. of supporters (= 100%)	47	29

in perceived burden associated with the sex or social class of the sup-porter, and the supporter's age appeared important only to the extent that 73% of supporters aged 25–44 reported no burden compared with 41% of those aged 45 and over. However one group of supporters – wives of the patients – was particularly prone to view the experience of caring as a large burden; 35% of wives said this compared with only 11% of other supporters. Only 12% of husbands said caring caused them a large burden, but their number was too small for this difference between the spouses to be statistically significant.

In other studies of carers the sex of both patients and carers, and the age of the carer, have been important factors (e.g. Zarit *et al.*, 1980; Gilleard *et al.*, 1984). However, many of these studies have looked at the supporters of the elderly mentally infirm, and the results are inconsistent. There has been some emphasis on the importance of the patient's moods or behavioural disturbance as a principal cause of burden (Greene *et al.*, 1982; Anderson, 1987); and it appears that among the stroke patients it is the patient's emotional and social behaviour, rather than physical dis-ability, which plays most part in influencing the experience of burden for the supporter. Wives appeared to be particularly sensitive to changes in relationship and the patient's personality. This probably enhances their perception of burden, as does the probability that they spent much time involved in caring for their husbands at home.

Coping by supporters

The burden of coping with stroke is only one part of the lives of supporters. The son of a woman who was living in a geriatric hospital noted:

You can cope with the old lady; it's just that you get other problems in your life which all contribute to physical and mental condition – my wife's illness, for example.

At the third interview all the supporters were asked whether anything had happened in their lives since the patient's stroke which made it more or less difficult for them to help the patient. Thirty-nine per cent of supporters referred to something which made it harder for them to help, most commonly that their own health had deteriorated; 10, or about a third, of these supporters said this. Supporters described worsening problems with both physical and mental health. The daughter of a woman who moved into sheltered housing explained:

I get more depressed. I've not got a lot of patience now. I feel guilty. I find I can't cope with things like I used to.

About half as many supporters identified problems in the health of others – their spouse's heart disease, angina or arthritis – which had made it more difficult to help the patient. Other family commitments and changes in work commitments were also identified as making it harder to support the patient.

On the other side, 29% of supporters identified things that had happened that made it easier for them to cope with helping the patient. These covered a more diverse range of events from having more time available (because they had changed jobs or retired) to the patient moving into sheltered or institutional care, and increased support from friends or welfare services.

One question which arises is whether, taking into account these changes and their current burden, supporters felt they were going to be able to cope in the future. Among supporters who felt that helping the patient caused any burden 18 months after the stroke 33% felt that in future they would need more help – that is, 17% of all supporters. The proportion who felt they would need more help included 18% of those who described the current burden as 'a little', 31% of those who said it was 'moderate', and 46% of those who described it as 'large'. Altogether, 29% of the supporters of male patients thought they were going to need more help compared with only 9% of the supporters of women. In the main, those who felt they were going to need help identified a probable need for more support from welfare services, such as the home help or bathing attendant, as well as respite care to give them a break or a holiday. The wife of a moderately disabled man noted:

I'm coping at the moment but you don't get a break or anything. It would be nice to go away for a holiday.

But another woman with a severely disabled husband commented:

It's just like having a family all over again. I have been debating, but what kind of help? I'll have to wait for the time to come. I don't think he would like anyone else around.

This concern about what is acceptable to the patient arises perhaps most sharply when supporters consider residential care for the patient. More than half of all supporters (53%) said they would be unable or unwilling to increase the amount of help they gave the patient – a feeling most pronounced among close female relatives (wife, daughter, sister), 62% of whom said this. This proportion was unrelated to the severity of the patient's residual disability, except that only 29% of the supporters of patients with no disability felt this, compared with 61% of the rest. Most clearly, only 14% of supporters who described the existing burden as moderate or large said they would be able to give more help, compared with 67% of those who felt there was no or just a little burden.

Supporters who did not feel willing or able to give 'a lot' more help were asked whether they would consider the stroke patient living in a home or long-stay hospital: 34% of this group said they would definitely consider this, 17% said possibly, 46% thought not and 3% did not know. So translated into proportions for all supporters, 19% would definitely consider residential care and 9% would possibly consider it. Only 14% of spouses of the patient said they would consider institutional care, but 38% of the patient's children acknowledged that they would consider this. Again, how the supporter felt about the existing burden was a clear guide to attitudes, insofar as 54% of the supporters who described the burden as moderate or large said they would consider institutional care, but only 13% of other supporters thought this. Finally, although supporters who lived with the patient appeared to experience more distressing consequences, few of them appeared to see institutional care as an alternative: only 9% of supporters who lived with the patient would consider this compared with 44% of the supporters of patients who lived in their own homes.

Preparation for coping with stroke

The diversity of problems and concerns among patients and their supporters offer considerable scope for providing information, but the data presented in previous chapters on help and support from hospital and community services indicate a deficit, due in part to lack of contact.

At their second interview, 9 months after the stroke, patients were asked whether they felt they had enough information about their illness and their recovery. Many had been confused and bewildered when first seen 3 or 4 weeks after the stroke, so it was both surprising and apparently reassuring to find that 77% of patients felt they had enough information and only 23% wanted more. However, the comments of patients who were 'satisfied' suggest that many had, in a fatalistic or resigned way, 'had enough' of stroke as well as any information about it:

I know what's wrong with me; there's no use discussing it with anybody – they can't help you.

I know what happened, as much as they can give. Dr Jones told me there's no treatment for me. Nothing can be done.

For other patients it appeared the experience was one they simply no longer wished to discuss:

No, I wouldn't want to know too much more. I don't want to know any more medical problems.

I'd like to forget all about it. I don't want to know more, as long as it doesn't come back.

The patients who felt they had had enough information were more likely to have been severely disabled after the stroke and to be aged 75 or over. The figures are shown in Table 67.

There were no differences in demand for information associated with the patient's sex or social class, nor with the hospital or ward type in which they were treated. Although the response of many of the patients who said they knew enough appeared to be defensive they were, as a group, neither more nor less emotionally distressed than other patients, nor did the responses of their supporters indicate they had higher levels of 'negative mood' or that they were a greater burden.

A quarter of the patients wanted more information about the stroke

Table 67. *Demand for further information at 9 months after the stroke related to patients' age and severity of disability at 1 month after stroke*

Severity of disability	Proportion of patients wanting more information about stroke/recovery		
	Age 60–74	Age 75 +	All patients
Very severe/severe	14% (14)[a]	6% (18)	9% (32)
Moderate/mild/none	45% (29)	17% (30)	31% (59)
All patients	35% (43)	13% (48)	23% (91)

[a] Figures in brackets are the numbers on which percentages are based.

and their recovery. As shown in Table 67, these were mainly younger patients with moderate or less severe disability. By far the most common question, even 9 months after the stroke, was 'Why me?'; almost half of these patients wanted to learn more about what caused their stroke:

You don't know what causes these strokes or anything about it. The doctors told me nothing.

I'd like to know the cause. You need a book for the layman: 'How to avoid a stroke'. [I asked in the hospital] doctor, sisters, but they didn't know.

Several patients linked their desire for information about causation to prospects for avoiding another stroke. A woman aged 62 who lived alone at home illustrates the dilemma she felt:

Well, I do think as to why it happened to me. I did ask the doctor when I went to hospital but gathered no one knows very much about strokes. If it had been a heart attack there are things you should and shouldn't eat; things you should and shouldn't do, but no one knows for stroke. People have in general said so little, I get the feeling if I knew what exercises to do it might help but no one seems to prescribe anything for a stroke. You see no one says to follow Lizzie in the morning [a keep-fit instructor on breakfast television] or, on the other hand, 'for God's sake don't attempt any violent exercise'.

Help and advice for carers

Supporters recall few helpful contacts with hospital staff. Although at 1 month after the stroke only 1 in 8 supporters reported receiving help or advice from the rehabilitation therapists, no other professional group in the hospital was mentioned more often.

Altogether, 37% of supporters said that someone had, in the month since the stroke, spoken with them about ways in which they might help

the patient get better or cope with his or her difficulties. This proportion
was not associated with the hospital or ward type. The supporters of older
patients were less likely to report receiving any advice: the proportion fell
from 52% among the supporters of patients aged 60–69, down to only
26% among the supporters of patients aged 80 or over. Possibly staff feel
that more might be achieved by involving the supporters of younger
patients; or perhaps the supporters of younger patients have more concerns about the future that they want to discuss with staff (though there
was no general relationship between age of the patient and the proportion
of supporters who were worried about how the patient would cope).

At their first interview fewer than 10% of supporters said they had
received advice from a nurse about how they could help the patient; and
about 5% that a hospital doctor had given advice to them. The few
contacts that supporters reported with doctors were mainly about practical help and prospects for the patient. A daughter explained she had seen
the consultant:

He said she's got to get a lot more confidence back – then she can get back to
normal. She has to take exercises. We went to the consultant because the young
ones didn't give us satisfaction.

Several of the supporters who had received no advice noted that they
too needed support and information from somebody. For example, the
wife of a man aged 63, who had been active in work and leisure before his
mild stroke, said:

Medically, it could have been explained to me better. More information is
required for the partner. It's my confidence that needs a help to encourage or
discourage activities.

And a daughter who lived a distance away but who was her mother's only
supporter observed:

I do feel there is still a painful lack of communication between the medical staff,
patients and their supporters. Sometimes you literally have to fight to get any
information; and it's extremely difficult to plan.

It may be argued that this picture of hospital support for the supporters
has been taken too soon, since at 1 month after the stroke a majority of
the patients were still in hospital. Supporters of patients who had been in
hospital were asked in their second interview, about 9 months after the
stroke, specifically about contacts with hospital doctors and nurses.
Although the proportion of supporters who reported contacts is about a
third for both doctors and nurses, the proportion of supporters who felt they
were given any helpful advice was only 1 in 10. The figures are in Table 68.

Table 68. *Supporters' views on help and advice from hospital doctors and nurses (9 months after the stroke)*

Since the stroke, supporter reports:	Hospital doctors (%)	Hospital nurses (%)
No contact	62	70
Contact, but no help or advice	21	20
Advice, but it was not helpful	5	1
Advice that was helpful	12	9
No. of supporters (= 100%)	85	85

So, in general, hospital doctors and nurses were not often seen by supporters as useful sources of help and advice. In part this reflects the organisation of care, which may not allocate time specifically for supporters, and which appears to involve supporters relatively little while the patient is in hospital. In part, too, once problems have been sorted out supporters may not recall all the advice they received. However, a major reason for the lack of impact by doctors and nurses is probably that neither group deals with the supporters' main worries and concerns – how they and the patients will cope at home in the future.

Patients and their supporters face different problems and have concerns which differ at the various stages after the stroke. Both groups have a persistent wish to understand something about the causes of the stroke, and what could be done to prevent another one. However, there are certain differences, for example in the way that the main concerns of the supporters changed over time: from anxieties about survival to concern about practical arrangements for the patients, and then to problems about their personal relationship with the patient and restrictions on their social life (Warlow *et al.*, 1987). At 18 months after the stroke it appeared that supporters were again increasingly concerned about the patient's physical dependency – a topic which appeared to be of enduring concern to the patients. These concerns and problems arose and were faced generally without specific advice from hospital or community staff, but at the first two interviews most patients and supporters expressed reasonable satisfaction with the amount and nature of information they received.

At the second interview two-thirds of the supporters said that they knew enough about the illness and that there was nothing more they wanted to know. However, at the third interview, 18 months after the stroke, 72% of supporters felt that, looking back, they had *not* been well prepared with advice or information for the problems they had had to face as a result of the stroke. Perhaps it was only when supporters judged that the patient's condition would improve no further that they also felt they should have been more aware of the potential difficulties. It is difficult for carers without previous experience of the illness to know what questions to ask; and it is only with hindsight that they can see they were not well prepared.

At the final interview supporters felt they should have been better informed in general terms:

Information about how such things are caused and might be avoided. What the psychological effects are likely to be. What the period of convalescence is likely to be. What prospects are there for a repetition? We go on in the dark.

They also wanted to have been told more about what to expect:

Nobody told me a thing about it, what to expect and what to do about it. Her diet. The things you get told are by people who've had people with strokes. It's the home help that's told us about things like getting the bed higher and the toilet seat.

They don't tell you anything; what it's like, what to expect. They don't even tell you what's wrong. I should have expected a social worker to make enquiries about how we're coping. They're not a bit helpful.

And they wanted to have been given information about benefits and services:

A more thorough breakdown of not only social benefits but financial, physical and otherwise provided by the DHSS. Information was bitty, half information.

You should be able to get on to somebody and find out what you should do. You get no answers from the doctor. There should be somewhere you could go. Someone that the doctor could say 'If you need help 'phone this number.'

Finally, they felt ill-prepared for the consequences of the stroke:

I would have liked things explained to me a bit. He was sent home and I was told he might get a bit depressed. They said he was quite self-sufficient. My goodness – I was not prepared for it.

I think it would have been nice to have known that she was going to change so completely, to a miserable old lady.

Although these comments were made 18 months after the stroke it is likely that supporters who face the unexpected or who are not prepared with knowledge about services find it harder to cope. The analyses suggest that it is the supporter who lives with the stroke patient who is most in need of this preparation and advice – and most of these supporters had the same general practitioner as the patient.

Assessments of recovery after stroke

In previous chapters changes in the lives of patients and supporters have been described, and some of their feelings about these changes have been discussed. Strokes clearly affect not only the health and physical capacity of patients but also the domestic habits, leisure activities and family relationships of both patients and their supporters. In the light of these changes, as well as the necessary re-organisation of work, housing and finances, what does it mean to talk of 'recovery' after a chronic illness? Health workers have usually viewed recovery as improvement in mobility and self-care and discharge from the medical or rehabilitation services. The question here is whether the same factors are given similar weight in the judgements of patients and their families about recovery from the stroke.

At each of the three interviews patients and supporters were asked how much recovery they felt the patient had made so far, and how much further improvement they expected. The pattern of responses changed over time, in part due to deaths of more seriously ill patients. Table 69 therefore only shows the views of the patients and supporters in each group who were seen at all three interviews.

For both patients and supporters these assessments, like the changes in levels of performance of activities, had changed most by the second interview, but the relative stability of the general pattern masks continuing, if lesser changes between the second and third interviews; for example the patients' assessment of recovery so far was constant in only 47% of cases and of recovery to be expected in 52% of cases. In general, assessments of the recovery that had been achieved declined only slightly over time, although the proportion of patients who felt they had made no recovery rose significantly from 4% at 1 month after the stroke to 18% at around 18 months. Expectations for recovery declined markedly over time for both patients and supporters, although at all stages supporters were less likely to think that the patients would make 'a lot' more recovery. By the third interview there was a high level of agreement between patient and supporter about how much recovery had been achieved (correlation of +0.51); but patients were much more likely to express continuing expectation for further recovery.

It is difficult to generalise about the meaning of recovery to patients and supporters although, as is the case with the main problems and

Table 69. *Views of patients and supporters on recovery achieved and expected*

Views of:	A lot	Some	Just a little	Not at all	No. of patients/ supporters (= 100%)
		Patient recovered			
Patients					
T1 (%)[a]	52	26	18	4	72
T2 (%)	42	31	16	11	75
T3 (%)	42	22	18	18	77
Supporters					
T1 (%)	50	22	22	6	72
T2 (%)	53	19	23	5	74
T3 (%)	42	25	21	12	75
		Patient expected to recover			
Patients					
T1 (%)	65	17	9	9	58
T2 (%)	27	27	27	19	67
T3 (%)	19	28	25	28	72
Supporters					
T1 (%)	35	36	21	8	61
T2 (%)	4	16	37	43	70
T3 (%)	1	1	30	68	74

[a] T1, 1 month after the stroke; T2, 9 months after the stroke; T3, 18 months after the stroke. Differences in base numbers are because some patients who responded at the third interview 18 months after the stroke were unable to answer at previous interviews.

concerns the two groups have, there appear to be differences between their views. Two approaches to considering these differences are used here: comparing statements about recovery, and looking at variables associated with the summary assessments of patients and supporters.

At the second interview half the patients, compared with a fifth of the supporters, were relatively optimistic about future improvement. They were helped in this by viewing recovery to that stage as 'relatively' good in relation to their age, to how they were immediately after the stroke, or to other patients.

One woman, who was becoming mobile at home in her wheelchair, commented about recovery so far:

Half-way there I should say. It's gradual. I'm very pleased really because I've seen some who were no different in the hospital to what they are now – stationary.

Another woman, who had been just a few weeks in hospital with a mild stroke, said of her recovery:

Well, it's going along slowly but the right way; I'm going on as well as anybody. Slow I think, but then they tell me it's a slow job. When I was in hospital I was walking as soon as I was out of bed, but some of them there were still in wheelchairs. I think I was lucky in some ways, but maybe it affected my brain box, that's what I call it, more than theirs.

At the other extreme a housebound woman commented that she had recovered:

Not an awful lot; I seem to have got worse. I'm not very happy about it at all. People older than me can get about but I don't get out at all.

In this phase, about 9 months after the stroke, most patients were viewing recovery in terms of how much they had achieved since the illness. They were often reinforced in this perspective by the comments of family and particularly of health service staff, whose main reference point is 'since the stroke'. Few patients, at this stage, judged recovery as 'being back to normal' – to how they were before the stroke. However, by the third interview 18 months after the stroke expectations of further recovery had fallen for most patients, and their supporters were considering a process which they felt was close to the end. In the following extracts the views of patients and supporters, interviewed independently, are presented together to illustrate differences in their perspectives. The comments have been selected on the basis of how typical they are of the patient's view.

At 18 months after the stroke the general picture presented by patients is of a recovery which has been slow and is seen particularly in terms of walking:

Well I have made some recovery but it seems to have slowed rapidly. I feel it's slow; I feel it could be more. To think I couldn't at one time and now I can hobble about.

The man's wife agreed:

He's made a good recovery; he couldn't walk or anything.

In this third interview patients put more emphasis on return to life as it was before the stroke. One woman reported:

I think I've got back to normal; just only the leg that aches when I walk on it.

But her daughter felt she had made 'just a little recovery' and emphasised the mental aspect of her mother's stroke:

Not a lot [of recovery]. She can move her hands now but she hasn't changed in temperament.

This inclination to include the mental and emotional consequences in their assessment of recovery is more typical of the supporters. One elderly woman reported:

I feel quite well. I don't feel I've got any effects from the stroke.

But her daughter-in-law's view was that:

Physically she's made a tremendous recovery, but mentally she is deteriorating.

For some patients, too, the emotional distress caused by the illness was a barrier to recovery. An ex-schoolteacher commented:

[Daughter] says I'm improving but I don't see how because if I was happy I wouldn't be as restless and upset. I think this business of being depressed is something outside myself and to do with the stroke. I reckon it's not part of me but to do with the stroke. I've got to think of the two things: my arthritis and my stroke. I find with this left hand I can hardly do the buttons.

In fact the daughter's view was similar, although it covered other issues. She felt her mother had improved:

Quite a bit. It took a long time and it's only in the last three months she's begun to get her speech, memory and writing improved. The hand doesn't seem to be improving.

As the last patient indicated, other illnesses may impede recovery from the stroke and be more important in the patient's daily life. A woman who was confined to the few steps between bed, chair and commode said of her recovery:

I haven't made any with this arthritis in the hand. I can't use it. I can't write hardly with the right hand. I'm hopeless, helpless.

Sadly, her son agreed:

She's got worse.

For patients, the key to their assessment of recovery appears to lie in what they are currently able to do, generally in terms of using an affected hand or walking. Often patients were happy simply to have finally repossessed some function. A man who was unable to walk at 1 month after the stroke said:

Let's put it this way; I started up I was going to recover, never any question of being like I was before. I feel it's very slow. I think I'm recovering but it's very slow indeed, particularly when you consider the time involved. I felt about the therapy it wasn't really putting anything in my pocket so to say. The usual way is to count your blessings. I can at least walk now with a stick which I couldn't before – very pleased about that.

This patient's wife similarly identified 'a lot' of improvement in performance although she felt it had stopped:

He's improved enormously from what he was when he first had it. The past few months has been more or less at a standstill.

From their comments it appears that patients were more concerned in the longer term about what they were able to do – essentially their physical performance – than whether they were doing well for their age or in comparison with other patients. The standards were more absolute than relative and, in the face of low expectations for further recovery, they were quite demanding. Supporters' views were generally similar to those of the patients, but they appeared to consider the mental and emotional elements of recovery more often. This is not surprising considering that they frequently viewed changes in the patient and in their relationship with the patient as a problem.

Factors influencing assessment of recovery

The second approach to considering what constitutes recovery lies in the analysis of other variables associated with assessments by patients and their supporters of how much recovery the patient had made. These analyses are discussed here for views of recovery over the 18 months following the stroke.

Patients

The assessments made by patients were hardly related to measures of change over time in physical disability. Table 70 shows that patients' views were not significantly associated with degree of improvement from 1 to 18 months after the stroke. A comparison with disability scores before the stroke distinguished only between those who felt they had recovered a lot and those who felt they had made less recovery.

Perception of recovery was more clearly associated with disability score at the time of the third interview than with change in disability score over time. The proportion of patients saying they had recovered a lot increased

Table 70. *Patients' assessments of their recovery related to their disability scores*

| Disability | Mean disability (change) score for patients who described their recovery as: | | | |
	A lot	Some	Just a little	Not at all
Change T0–T3[a]	−1.6	−3.8	−3.6	−4.0
Change T1–T3	+2.5	+2.5	+2.7	+1.0
Barthel score at T3	17.3	15.1	14.4	13.4
No. of patients	32	17	14	14

[a]T0, before the stroke; T1, 1 month after the stroke; T3, 18 months after the stroke.

from 9% of those with a score of 6 or less to 56% of patients with a disability score of 15 or 16. So the lack of association between changes in disability and perception of recovery reflects the finding that patients with greater disability achieve a greater change in disability score. Put another way, of patients classified at the third interview as having mild disability or no disability on the Barthel index, 53% felt they had made 'a lot' of recovery, compared with only 17% of patients who were classified as having moderate or severe disability.

Characteristics of the stroke – such as whether or not it was a first stroke, whether there was a speech problem, and the side of weakness – were not associated with the patient's assessment of recovery, nor were measured changes in housework or social activities. However, certain social characteristics of the patient – age, marital status and social class, but not sex, home ownership or household size – were clearly associated with perception of recovery.

Older patients were more likely to feel they had made no recovery; the proportion saying this increased from 5% of patients aged 60–69, to 40% of those aged 80 or over. Again this seems to reflect differences in current performance, since there were no significant differences by age in physical recovery from before the stroke to the third interview. The patient's social class clearly distinguished perspectives on recovery: only 19% of patients classified as middle-class felt they had recovered a lot compared with 48% of working-class patients. This may reflect expectations among middle-class patients which were not tapped in general questions (for example plans for the future), or it may be that middle-class patients somehow felt they were more handicapped; it was not because they were any more disabled, but it does parallel the finding reported in Chapter 5 that middle-class patients were more likely to regard their disabilities as a problem.

There appears to be an effect of home, particularly marital, relationships on assessment of recovery. Altogether only 27% of married patients felt they had made 'a lot' of recovery compared with 54% of patients who were widowed. Even among patients with mild or no disability at the third interview only 33% of married patients compared with 68% of widowed patients described their recovery as 'a lot'. There were no differences in perception of recovery associated with household size, but assessments were related to patients' views on household relationships: 52% of those who described their relationships as very happy felt they had recovered a lot, compared with 18% of patients who felt relationships at home were only fairly happy or not very happy.

Specifically, among those who described their marital relationships as very happy, 47% said they had recovered a lot compared with only 9% of other patients. There was no such association between assessments of recovery and quality of relationships with children. It is difficult to say whether quality of marriage affects assessment of recovery or whether both are related to some other causal factor – probably both influence each other. But, among patients who felt they had recovered a lot, only 9% identified any problem for their spouse caused by the stroke compared with 27% of patients who felt they had made less recovery.

Supporters

The generally high level of agreement between the views about recovery of patients and supporters is reflected in the variables which appear to influence a supporter's assessment of recovery. Supporters of married patients were more likely to see little recovery: 47% described recovery as 'little' or 'not at all' compared with only 24% of the supporters of other patients. Accordingly, 52% of the spouses of stroke patients felt the patient had recovered 'little' or 'not at all' compared with only 23% of other supporters. There was, however, no difference in the supporters' assessments of recovery between those who did and did not live with the patient.

The patient's performance of activities of daily living, and change in disability, has an important effect on supporters' views, as Table 71 shows. Supporters' views on recovery were consistently associated with disability scores at the third interview: there was a steady increase in the proportion of patients described as recovering 'a lot', from 18% of those

Table 71. *Supporters' assessment of the patient's recovery related to disability score*

| | Recovery at 18 months | | | |
Disability	A lot	Some	Just a little	Not at all
Change T0–T3[a]	−1.8	−2.5	−4.1	−5.9
Change T1–T3	+1.9	+1.9	+2.4	+0.2
Barthel score at T3	16.6	15.2	14.4	10.9
No. of supporters	30	19	16	9

[a] T0, before the stroke; T1, 1 month after the stroke; T3, 18 months after the stroke.

classified as severely disabled on the Barthel index to 65% of those classified as normal.

Changes in disability score were associated with assessments of recovery, but only when life before the stroke was taken as the reference point ($r = 0.37$). The extent to which patients make functional improvement after the stroke does not appear to be an important factor discriminating the assessments of either the patients or the supporters.

Satisfaction with recovery

For both patients and supporters, views on how much the patient had recovered and how satisfied they were with the recovery were strongly related: satisfaction with recovery was rated using the FACES scale, in which respondents identify their attitudes with one of a series of faces (Andrews and Withey, 1976) labelled A (the most positive) to G (the most negative). Among patients who felt they had made 'a lot' of recovery, 80% rated recovery as A or B, compared with 13% of other patients; among supporters who felt the patient had made 'a lot' of recovery 65% rated this A or B, compared with 10% of other supporters. The distribution of ratings by patients and supporters is shown in Table 72.

Although the distribution of responses to this question on satisfaction is similar for patients and supporters, individual patients and their supporters did not usually agree exactly with each other. When there were views from both sources they agreed in 16% of cases and 47% were within one grade of each other. The views of patients and their supporters are, therefore, presented independently in the analysis in order to identify

Table 72. *Ratings of recovery by patients and supporters*

FACES scale		Patients (%)	Supporters (%)
A		17	16
B		26	19
C		21	21
D		13	14
E		11	14
F		6	8
G		6	8
No. of patients or supporters		70	71

what factors influenced their judgements about the quality of the patient's recovery.

As response groups, those choosing faces A and B are clearly positive, happy or satisfied, while those choosing faces E, F or G are to varying extents disappointed and dissatisfied. In general, these two groups have been used as a basis for discriminating the responses of patients and of supporters.

Patients

There are few variables that clearly distinguished between patients who were either more satisfied or less satisfied with their recovery. The clearest difference was related to current level of disability; again the extent of improvement in disability score since the stroke was not important, but patients who remained moderately or severely disabled more than 1 year after the stroke were less satisfied with their recovery. None of the patients with severe or moderate disability identified their recovery with face A and 47% chose faces E, F or G; the corresponding proportions for patients with mild or no disability were 24% and 14%.

Patients who felt they did things socially, with other people, much less than they had done before the stroke were least likely to be positive about their recovery (only 9% identified recovery with faces A or B, compared with 61% of others). Also the level of their current social activities was clearly related to satisfaction with recovery: the proportion of patients who rated their recovery as A or B was 27% of those scoring 11 or less on the index of social activities, but increased to 82% of those scoring 16 or more. Patients' perception of change in themselves as people was also a consideration: only 7% of those who felt they had changed in themselves rated their recovery as A, compared with 28% of the patients who felt they were no different as a person.

Attitudes to recovery were not consistently associated with the patient's age, social class or household composition. However, married patients appeared to be disappointed with their recovery more often: 30% of them felt their recovery was represented by faces E, F or G, compared with only 9% of widowed patients.

Supporters

Supporters' feeling about the recovery were associated clearly only with the patient's disability score and with the supporters' own views on the quality of their relationship with the patient. The proportion of supporters who rated recovery as A or B was 54% among those who at 18 months after the stroke described their relationship with the patient as very happy, but fell to 27% of those who said it was fairly happy and to none of those who felt it was not very happy. The patient's age, sex and social class did not appear to be important, nor did the supporter's formal relationship to the patient (wife, son, etc.), or whether the supporter lived with the patient. However, the supporters' attitudes to recovery were related to the patient's current disability, particularly for those supporters who were disappointed: the proportion who rated recovery with faces E, F or G fell from 64% of supporters of patients who were severely or very severely disabled to only 6% of supporters of patients who were classified as normal on the Barthel index.

There therefore appears to be a consistent pattern among supporters as to the factors that affect their views on the extent of the patient's recovery and how satisfied they are with it. None of the standard demographic variables (sex, age or social class of supporters) was associated with their satisfaction with recovery.

Enjoyment of, and satisfaction with, life

In many senses the ultimate concern of this research is what difference having a stroke made to the quality of life of patients and their supporters. The issue has been addressed by looking at changes in patterns of living and at various measures of the impact of stroke – on emotional distress, family relationships and social involvements – but there was an opportunity to ask directly at the third interview for the global view of patients and supporters as to how the stroke had affected their enjoyment of life.

Altogether 36% of patients said they were enjoying life much less than they had before the stroke, and 35% said they were enjoying life slightly less. No patient said life was more enjoyable since the stroke. The views of patients and supporters were related ($r = 0.25$), although 45% of supporters thought there had been no change in their enjoyment of life. The association between the views of patients and their supporters is shown in Table 73, which indicates that 42% of the supporters of those patients who said they were enjoying life much less since the stroke also described changes in their own enjoyment of life in the same way.

Male patients were markedly more likely to report that they were enjoying life much less: more than half (52%) said this compared with only 27% of women. In their comments several of the men referred to a loss of freedom or independence – themes which hardly cropped up in the responses of women patients. Since the social lives of the men appeared

Table 73. *Views of patients and their supporters about how much they enjoy life now compared with before the stroke*

Supporter enjoys life	Patients' enjoyment of life			
	Much less (%)	Slightly less (%)	No change (%)	All supporters (%)
Much less	42	25	17	27
Slightly less	29	20	22	25
No change	25	50	61	45
More	4	5	0	3
No. of supporters (= 100%)	24	20	18	75

no more or less disrupted than those of the women it may be that this feeling of loss of freedom draws upon a more general sense of loss in the lives of men who, in the years before the stroke, had been used to involvement in work and contacts outside the home. There may also be some sense of loss of control, or power, in the home, and it seems likely that this difference is associated with a different experience of stroke for married patients: half the married patients reported enjoying life much less compared with only a quarter of the widowed patients. Perhaps married patients felt they had lost more of their future as well as of their current relationships.

In general, changes in physical disability were not consistently related to views about changes in enjoyment of life. There was no relationship with changes in disability scores since the stroke, and changes relative to the situation before the stroke were again only important in general terms, distinguishing those patients who were more disabled (47% of whom said they were enjoying life much less) from those patients who had returned to or (slightly) improved upon their disability score for life before the stroke (21% of whom said they were enjoying life much less). Similarly a patient's Barthel score at the third interview only distinguished between those with the maximum score (17% of whom said they enjoyed life much less) and those with any disability (43% of whom reported enjoying life much less than they had done before the stroke).

Changes in enjoyment of life reported by patients were not associated with the patient's age or social class, nor were the views of supporters associated with these characteristics of the patient. However, 68% of the supporters of male patients said they were enjoying life less compared with 41% of the supporters of women patients; and 70% of the supporters of married patients were enjoying life less compared with 40% of the supporters of other patients. Characteristics of the stroke – including side of weakness, loss of speech, incontinence and whether it was a first or subsequent stroke – were not associated with changes in enjoyment of life. As regards disability, supporters of patients classified as having no disability 18 months after the stroke were less likely to report a major reduction in enjoyment of life (6% did) than were supporters of patients who were rated as disabled to some degree, 33% of whom felt that their life was much less enjoyable.

Altogether, changes in the supporters' enjoyment of life appeared to be influenced at least as much by the person with the stroke as by the impairment as such. It is difficult to disentangle these variables, but it appears to be the supporter's relationship to the patient that is most important. First, there is a major difference between spouses of patients and other supporters in the proportion who described life as less enjoyable: 78% of spouses said this compared with 37% of others. But this is principally a difference associated with being the wife of the patient, among whom 85% reported that life was less enjoyable. Altogether there was no significant difference between male and female supporters in reported changes in enjoyment. The key general factor influencing change in enjoyment of life appears to be neither the patient's sex nor the supporter's sex, but whether the patient and supporter were living together at the time of the third interview. This is shown in Table 74, which also presents the differences by sex of the supporters and patient. Supporters who lived with the patient were considerably more likely than others to report that they enjoyed life less, but sex differences between supporters who did and did not live with the patient were not consistently significant.

A further important variable appears to be the supporter's view of the quality of the relationship between supporter and patient before the stroke. While only 42% of supporters who described the relationship before the stroke as very happy were enjoying life less, this proportion was 69% among supporters who said the relationship had been only fairly happy or not happy. It was among the supporters of patients who lived separately in their own homes that the quality of the relationship before the stroke was a decisive factor: only 11% of those who had enjoyed a very happy relationship reported that, at 18 months after the stroke, they enjoyed life less, compared with 63% of the rest.

The feeling that social life was restricted by the stroke appeared to contribute strongly to the supporter's view that life was less enjoyable

Table 74. *Proportion of supporters who enjoy life less after the stroke,
related to whether or not they live with the patient*

	Supporter lives with patient		
	Yes	No	All supporters
Supporter's sex:			
Male	60% (10)[a]	17% (12)	36% (22)
Female	91% (22)	35% (31)	58% (53)
Patient's sex:			
Male	85% (20)	36% (11)	68% (31)
Female	75% (12)	28% (32)	41% (44)
All supporters	81% (32)	30% (43)	52% (75)

[a] Figures in brackets are the numbers on which percentages are based.

since the stroke. Altogether 27% of supporters described life as much less
enjoyable and 25% reported that it was slightly less so; but the proportion
of supporters who felt life was either much less or slightly less enjoyable
increased from 24% of those who felt their life was 'not at all' restricted to
93% of those who felt that the stroke had 'severely' restricted their social
life.

The proportion of supporters enjoying life less increased with age, from
27% of those aged 25–44 to 70% of those aged 65 and over, but this trend
was a product of the increased likelihood that older supporters lived with
the patient. There were no social class differences among supporters in
their reports of changes in enjoyment of life. Clearly many factors mediate
the effects of stroke on the life of the supporter. Living with the patient,
the quality of the relationship with the patient before the stroke, and
changes in the supporter's opportunities to maintain a social life appear
to be major considerations.

SUMMARY

Caring From the time of the stroke most supporters regarded themselves as being the primary source of help and support for patients.
However, in the interviews 1 month after the stroke nearly three-quarters
of the supporters expressed worries about helping the patient – particularly about conflict with other commitments and about whether the
patient could be looked after properly. At 18 months after the stroke

nearly half the supporters said they were then spending much more time helping with practical jobs, and people living with the patient were more likely to say this. Altogether two-thirds of supporters who had increased their practical help said it caused them problems, most commonly tiredness. This was not simply a product of the patient's disability, and none of the supporters described giving the practical help, as such, as a great problem. However, supporters were, in general, reluctant to describe the help they gave as a problem. The supporters concept of burden seemed to be related to time constraints and difficulties with the patient as a person, rather than to the tasks that had to be done. At 18 months after the stroke one-third of supporters described the burden of caring as moderate or large. This proportion was higher among the supporters of emotionally distressed patients but, among patients with disability, it was not related to the severity of the disability. Two aspects of life before the stroke appeared to influence the supporters' feelings of burden: the quality of their relationship with the patient, and their assessment of their health. After the stroke three particular problems caused most distress: the patient's physical dependency, social restrictions on the supporter, and the patient's negative moods. Wives appeared to be particularly sensitive to changes in the patient as a person and (as seen in the previous chapter) to feeling that their social lives were restricted; they were most likely to experience caring as a large burden.

Coping with stroke   During the 18 months of the study the lives of the supporters changed in many ways that affected their capacity for coping with problems caused by the stroke. At the final interview a third of those experiencing some burden felt that they would need more help in the future – from social services but also respite care. More than half of all supporters said they would be unable or unwilling to increase the amount of help they gave the patient, and more than a quarter of the supporters said that they would consider residential care; this latter proportion was higher among the children than among the spouses of patients, and fewer than a tenth of the supporters who were living with the patient said they would consider institutional care.

In the first few weeks following the stroke many patients were confused and uncertain; by 9 months after the stroke most (three-quarters) felt they knew enough about it. Many of the patients, however, indicated that they had simply 'had enough' of stroke as well as of talk about it. The patients with a continuing demand for information tended to be younger and to have moderate or less severe disability. The most common question was still 'Why me?'

Few of the supporters reported any helpful contact with hospital staff; only 1 in 10 of them said they had received any helpful advice or instruction from either the nurses or the doctors in hospital. Among patients and, more sharply, among supporters the main concerns and anxieties changed over time. However, reasonable satisfaction with information was expressed until the final interview (at which time the physical recovery is basically over), when nearly three-quarters of the supporters felt that they had not been well prepared for the problems resulting from the stroke.

Assessments of recovery   Expectations for recovery declined markedly over time among both patients and supporters, although at all stages supporters were less likely to expect 'a lot' more recovery. Their assessments about the extent of the patient's recovery changed relatively little over time. At 18 months after the stroke 42% of both groups felt the patient had made 'a lot' of recovery. However, the proportion of patients who felt they had made no recovery increased from 4% at 1 month after the stroke to 18% at 18 months. The standards by which patients and supporters evaluated recovery changed over time, although for patients the ability to walk and to perform activities of daily living appeared to be consistently most important. Supporters' views were generally similar to the patients', but they were more likely to incorporate considerations about the mental and emotional condition of the patient. Married and middle-class patients were less likely to feel they had made a good recovery. The patient's disability at 18 months after the stroke was associated with the views of both patients and supporters about the extent of, and satisfaction with, recovery; but the amount of functional improvement since the stroke was not generally important in this respect.

Enjoyment of life   Thirty-six percent of patients and 27% of supporters reported that they were enjoying life much less since the stroke. Male patients and their supporters were more likely to say this. Among supporters, those who lived with the patient, and especially wives of patients, were more likely to be enjoying life much less. In general, relationships before the stroke and the problems caused by the stroke were a more significant determinant of satisfaction with life than were measures of disability. At 18 months after the stroke only half of either the patients or the supporters described themselves as hopeful about the patient's future.

CHAPTER NINE

Resources for coping with stroke

This book has sought to describe and illuminate the experiences and attitudes of stroke patients and their carers. It looks at the meaning of the illness for the everyday lives of those affected; it reflects the reality of a life-threatening condition of sudden onset, which may shatter personal images, family life and future ambitions. There has been a serious gap in our knowledge of coping with stroke from the perspectives of patients and carers rather than from that of medical and other service providers. Yet a sound, effective and ethical approach to stroke must lie in awareness of and attention to the experiences, values, priorities and expectations of patients and their carers – they are the people who live with the consequences of the illness and who shoulder its burdens.

Like all chronic illnesses, stroke represents an assault upon many areas of everyday life, and, as the results of the study reported here show, the nature and extent of the problems change over time since onset of the illness. These events are worked through in an environment which differs for each patient, with variations in the important resources of family, money, housing, health care and other services. In addition, the activities and performance of the people involved – patient, family, therapists, doctors – affect each other, so that in this complexity it is impossible to predict the experience of any individual patient. However, there are some common elements in the experience of the people studied here, and some distinctive differences between particular groups. These are discussed in the next section before going on to consider the implications of results from this research for policy and practice. The circumstances in Greenwich Health District at the time of the study were not outstandingly better or worse than elsewhere in the United Kingdom, but there are large variations between districts in resources and practices which will determine the detailed specifications for the more general proposals outlined here. The patients and their carers in this study are in many ways typical of the older people who suffer the aftermath of a stroke; this record of their expectations, satisfactions, frustrations and fears offers a new picture of their life in the first year and a half after the illness.

The experience of stroke

Patients and carers suffer from a variety of interlocking social, emotional, economic and physical problems. This points towards the need for an integrated perspective, and practice, to understand and respond to the experience. The orientation towards a psychosocial rather than a medical model of illness has been widely canvassed (Engel, 1977; Illsley, 1980) and clearly is more appropriate to the experience of patients, at least after the very early phase of emergency medical care. Nearly all the energy applied to improving the situation after stroke is directed to making changes in levels of functioning (disability) and minimising social or economic disadvantage (handicap); very little is done to address neurophysiological losses (impairments). Of course, these different levels of disablement are linked, particularly severity of impairment and physical disability. It was much less clear that the severity of physical disability had a major effect on the quality of experience in other areas of life or that the physical aspects of care were the most important to supporters.

The severity of the disability is significant for the patient's response to and experience of the illness (affecting expectations, attitudes to rehabilitation, use of services and length of hospital stay), but it appears less important as an influence on everyday activities. Patients rated as having no disability (and their supporters) reported many of the same problems as the more disabled patients. This probably reflects some distress caused by having the illness at all, as well as the fairly low level of performance that is classified as independence on the Barthel index. The lack of a relationship between severity of the condition and handicap or disadvantage has been observed for conditions such as heart disease (Mayou, 1986) as well as for stroke (Christie, 1982), and it accords with common clinical experience. In the case of stroke it has been suggested (Hyman, 1972; Christie, 1982) that social and psycological factors conditioning response to rehabilitation may have an important influence on the relationship between different levels of disablement. Among the patients we studied those who were emotionally distressed and socially isolated appeared to make less recovery, in the sense of improvement in physical functioning. Attitudes to the illness and to disability appear to have a ubiquitous influence on response to the stroke and its consequences: though, of course, some people cope better than others with crises and dilemmas. The problem, however, is that these attitudes to illness and disability, although recognised as potentially critical for recovery (Andrews and Stewart, 1979; Henley *et al.*, 1985), are so often seen as personality characteristics, such as 'motivation', when they are in practice mutable and respond to a variety of conditions, possibly including counselling.

Among both patients and carers there appear to be relatively high levels of emotional distress associated with the stroke, although this takes many forms, such as depression, anxiety and emotional lability (Warlow *et al.*, 1987). Depressed mood is often persistent after the stroke (Wade *et al.*, 1987) and among Greenwich patients the presence of emotional distress was remarkably constant over the 18 months after the stroke. However, like other aspects of response to the illness, it seems that the patient's mental state changes over time from initial confusion and disorientation, through more active distress or frustration, towards resignation and acceptance. The whole process may take years and, as Holbrook (1982) points out, a significant proportion of patients may reject the idea that they could ever accept their condition. From the perspective of carers, the patient's mood and mental state usually moved in a negative direction, and appeared to cause particular problems during the second half of the first year after the stroke.

Some differences between patients and carers

For most patients and their carers the stroke led to a marked deterioration in enjoyment of, and feelings of satisfaction with, life. However, the experience of living with stroke is different in many respects for patients and carers: different problems are important for them at different stages following the stroke and they have different perspectives on outcome. The problems of coping with stroke change over time although at each stage the social and psychological problems were mentioned by carers as often as any physical difficulties – and this appears to be true in general for the carers of people with chronic illness (Anderson, 1987). There are clear implications for continuity of support, and some indications that patients and their carers who live together should be a priority group for social and welfare services, especially if relationships before the stroke were not good.

In some ways the stroke was more threatening to the carers than to the stroke patients. Carers had more worries early on about problems such as housing and the patient's mental health, and they were more actively engaged in looking for strategies to deal with the consequences of the illness. They tended to view changes as having been more dramatic and were more sensitive to changes in the patient as a person, and in their relationship together. This is probably a product, in part, of the greater insight available to some carers as well as a reflection of the knowledge that they themselves will often not only live with the illness as much as do the patients but will feel more responsibility, as well as more uncertainty, about coping with the stroke.

Carers do not usually suffer equivalent physical restrictions, although many are elderly themselves, but they may be caught up in the patient's web of social and economic problems. Patients often appeared to reorganise their values in their experience of, and expectations of, daily life – so, for example, 'comfort' could become more important than 'activity', and having few social activities outside the family could be accommodated. They could accept more modest aspirations and ambitions as the only feasible strategy for coping with the disruption to their lives. Carers, on the other hand, frequently had other work and family commitments; more than half were from a generation younger than the patient, so it was probably harder for many of them to legitimate and accept this major upset to their plans. For carers of the same generation the loss was often deepened because the patient was their main companion and partner; they not only felt tied, restricted or unable to pursue interests but, in more than half the cases, they felt that the person with whom they had shared experiences was no longer the same. This is not to say that the experience of stroke was somehow worse for carers, though for some it evidently was. Taken altogether, patients had higher levels of emotional distress than carers, although they were not much more satisfied or dissatisfied with 'life as a whole' (Anderson, 1988).

The general conclusion is that the experience of stroke is different for patients and their carers as regards attitudes, expectations, health and changes in daily life. Both groups are profoundly affected by the event but in different ways at different times with, consequently, different needs for information and support. The severity of the stroke, and of the disability, provides a useful guide to the prospects for physical recovery but gives little indication of how the lives of patients and carers will be affected.

Variations among carers

The main factors influencing the experience of carers appeared to be related to whether the carer lived with the patient and to the quality of the carer's relationship with the patient before the stroke, rather than to characteristics of the stroke. Because of the relatively small numbers in the study it is difficult to disentangle the main variables, but it seems that women carers, and particularly wives (the main group living with the patients), were more adversely affected by the stroke than were male carers.

The wives of patients identified more problems associated with the stroke than others; they, and other women, were more likely than male carers to report stress and deleterious effects on health (mainly worry, exhaustion and mental strain), and they were more likely to feel their life had changed and been restricted by the stroke. More of the women than men carers felt that the increasing help they gave caused them problems, although few of them reported that physical or domestic work was a major issue. It may be that women are more sensitive to changes in the patient as a person, more distressed by the effects of the illness on their personal relationship and by their loss of companionship and, perhaps (Arber *et al.*, 1988), more likely to be, or to feel, left alone by family and services to cope with problems. In several ways the phrase 'only the wife knows' may be true. However, their experience of some of the worst consequences was not translated into expressions of burden or greater preparedness to consider institutional care. Perhaps there is considerable cultural taboo against a caring wife admitting either of these feelings (Finch, 1989).

Sex, age and social class of patients

It was consistently difficult to tell whether this experience of women carers was due to a charateristic common to the carers, to the patients or to the relationship between them. In some ways men may be more difficult patients: they were not more disabled, nor did they report more emotional distress, but they were more likely to feel they were enjoying life 'much less' since the stroke, and more of them than seemed merited by their physical disability felt unable to look after themselves in some way. A group of 'disappointed' or even 'embittered' men was noticeable among the younger (under 75) patients. Several had been in employment or recently retired with good reason to be looking forward to years of 'well-earned leisure'. The stroke caused a disruption of plans for the future, a loss of freedom or independence and probably, too, some revision of relationships at home, particularly with wives. It is likely that this response among some men made life more difficult for their caring spouses, who had also seen plans for the future dashed and their relationships transformed. This conjecture needs further research, but whatever the reason, women caring at home for their husbands appear to be a group whose health and quality of life is seriously at risk following the stroke.

Younger patients were more likely to have been living with a spouse, or someone else at home before the stroke. In some ways younger people seemed more inclined to view the stroke as a drama and disruption in their lives: they were more likely to go straight to hospital rather than call a doctor; they were less satisfied with the information that they received about their illness; and although they were more likely to regain the (measured) functional abilities that they had before the stroke, they were more likely to feel their mobility had declined and to give up more of their social activities. There may be several explanations for these findings, but older patients may find it easier to view the stroke as part of the ageing process and to accommodate it more easily. Nevertheless, there is a very fine line between despondency and coping well; if older people somehow modified their expectations and lived with less hope for recovery and for life in general, this was not reflected in the assessments of their emotional state or enjoyment of life.

Three-quarters of the patients were classified as working-class. Not surprisingly, category of social class was not associated with the severity or nature of the impairment after the stroke, but it did seem to influence the patient's actions and reaction to the illness. There was a social class gradient in the direct use of hospital casualty departments such that a large proportion of working-class patients went straight to hospital without contacting their doctor and, in the longer-term, fewer of the working-class patients had seen their general practitioner. It seems likely that previous experience of unsatisfactory health care in the area (LHPC, 1981) made some contribution to differences in help-seeking among working-class patients. In other ways, such as adequacy of housing and money, it could be expected that middle-class patients would be better off. However, there were no differences in ratings of the suitability of housing – although this could be due, in part, to the take-up of well-equipped sheltered housing by working-class, but not middle-class, patients. In general, patients classified as middle-class were more likely to view the illness as having a damaging effect on themselves and their lives: more of them felt lonely; fewer of them felt they had made 'a lot' of recovery; more of them viewed their dependency as a problem; and, as a group, middle-class patients rated themselves as less satisfied with life (Anderson, 1988). Again this may reflect a greater sense of loss among people who before the stroke had more choice and control in their daily lives.

The social patterning of responses to the stroke shows how the meaning and significance of the illness is influenced by the context in which it occurs and the expectations or aspirations of the people involved. Clearly physical independence is only one of several possible goals for patients and possibly not the ultimate objective of most, or of their carers for them. A large number of patients focus their ambitions on walking and using their hands but many are not preoccupied by this, including some who were restricted in mobility or self-care before the stroke. It would probably be appropriate to view independence less in terms of doing mundane physical tasks and more in relation to the ability to make personal, social and economic choices. Seen from this perspective, the goal is not to achieve or carry out the maximum number of tasks without help, but the quality of life and of human relationships that can be achieved with assistance. Needing or giving help with mobility or self-care, for example, can thus be seen as less important than being unable to occupy time effectively, or to maintain social relationships. A key skill for patients may be learning to accept help from others rather than striving to perform all tasks themselves.

The values and expectations of patients and carers are affected by variables such as social position, age, personality and severity of disability, but also probably by more tangible and modifiable conditions such as level of knowledge and awareness about stroke, quality of contact with health workers, and relevant support at home and in the community – which is where 6 out of 7 survivors live.

Help and support from services

The appropriateness of services should be seen in terms of the extent to which they meet the needs and preferences of patients and carers; and the extent to which limited resources are concentrated effectively around the problems that matter to patients and carers (which will usually, but not always, include survival).

Communication with patients and carers

One important need that was consistently identified, particularly by its absence, was the need for information. Patients and carers are anxious for knowledge in quite explicit areas: causation of the stroke and risk of recurrence; prognosis and rate of recovery; mental health and social isolation; services available and what they can do to help themselves. These concerns are predictable and widely acknowledged by professionals, who recognise different needs of patients and carers; probably fewer, though, realise how these needs for information change over time.

This awareness was not translated into a systematic effort to inform. In particular, a majority of carers felt they had been ill-prepared for the events and experiences that followed the stroke.

The provision of timely and effective communication is difficult since needs will depend upon individual circumstances and preferences, while the future for individual patients is not generally entirely predictable. However, advice, information, support and encouragement should be at the centre of strategies to enhance the quality of life of patients and their carers. The focus of services cannot be upon the repair of underlying physical damage or even on remedial therapy; it needs to be committed on a continuous basis to improving education and training for living with chronic illness. This implies better education and training for service providers: so that nurses, for example, can become more sensitive to the needs and experiences of patients; so that staff can listen and talk together with patients and their carers, identifying preferences for information (acknowledging that some patients, especially those who are older and more disabled, may not wish to cope with too much information) and preferences for caring. There is a need for service providers to recognise differences between their perceptions and those of others if they are to bridge the existing gaps in communication.

Patients and carers in the early phase hope for and expect significant recovery from the stroke, but neither group appears to expect miracles. They believe that rehabilitation services can help them, but seem to feel that, in the community, there is not a lot that doctors can do. The general practitioners appear to play a relatively limited role in the continuing support of patients and seem to be involved even less with carers. Yet the general practitioner has, in principle, an important contribution to make as the doctor offering 'continuing care' sensitive to psychological aspects (House *et al.*, 1989) and as perhaps the only professional who is at all knowledgeable about the problems of both patient and carer. General practitioners could respond to the main expressed need – for 'caring interest' – as well as being in a good position to provide timely information. Even 9 months after the stroke a quarter of the patients in the community were apparently unaware of their diagnosis of stroke and, although no longer bewildered, many still did not understand why the illness had happened or what the implications were for recovery. Carers have a more extensive range of concerns but had seldom talked with any caring professional about them, and only exceptionally to hospital doctors and nurses.

Co-ordinated care in the community

The management of a chronic illness, such as stroke, demands a leading contribution from services in the community, particularly those in primary health care, with their orientation to family care and continuity of care (Cartwright, 1967; Cartwright and Anderson, 1981). The disability caused by chronic illness has been described as 'the very stuff of general practice' (Hasler, 1985), yet there are significant reports of unclear responsibilities, poor co-ordination and inadequate communication within and between general practice and other elements of the services (Blaxter, 1976; Royal College of Physicians, 1986). Perhaps these problems reflect an overemphasis upon the general practitioner as the natural leader, co-ordinator and strategist, at the expense of contributions from others in the primary health care team. Many of the doctors in the study said they would like to do more themselves for their stroke patients, and they often articulated the main longer-term problems clearly, but they did not appear to take the corresponding initiative in contacts with patients and carers (see also in Warlow *et al.*, 1987). Perhaps patients should be given their discharge notes when they leave hospital and advised to discuss their experience with the general practitioner, preferably in their own home.

The nature of the longer-term management of stroke in the community – providing information, caring interest and effective liaison with diverse health and social agencies – does not dictate that the general practitioner should have the key role within primary health care; it may be equally acceptable and more practical to train community nurses in counselling and the other skills necessary to support their client groups. However, as Twigg and colleagues (1990) point out, the potential of community nursing, or other services, will only be realised if services are organised more specifically. Commitment to help and its continued availability are the key elements; it is probably much less important to patients and carers who takes the lead, than that they reliably have someone to relate to. The identity of the 'key' contact is probably more important to the different professional groups who will co-ordinate their various contributions in health, social, domestic and rehabilitation services.

The co-ordination of care teams has proved difficult to structure and the potential for such teams will be very different in different areas. However, there is no real alternative: the idea of a 'generic' worker with skills drawn from different team members is still promoted (Royal College of Physicians, 1990) but appears to be a non-starter with the different professions. Thus, the prospects for improved stroke services will depend upon systems to increase flexibility and co-operation among the caring professions, as well as training to expand awareness of both problems and opportunities.

Among the individual services the performance of the social and domestic services appeared relatively satisfactory, although there were often grumbles about standards. On the whole these services reached those who needed and wanted them most, and this was also a finding of a study in the Bristol area (Legh-Smith, 1986). Use of home helps and Meals on Wheels was, as is generally the case (Social Services Inspectorate, 1987), associated with living alone, but not with the sex of the carer nor generally with the severity of the disability. The bathing service did not seem to be highly targeted on those most in need, but few wanted more of this. The most common need, as shown also in other studies, was for improved chiropody services (Cartwright and Henderson, 1986).

Most of the help and support for patients was coming from family and friends, typically from one main carer, not from services; and while most of the carers were coping with the practical caring tasks, many identified a need for support from social services to sort out housing and financial problems. The provision of more continuing interest and support for dealing with these social problems should contribute to easing the 'burden' on the carers, although there remains a need for co-ordination of planned respite care and arrangements for free time. Above all, the burden and stress of caring would be relieved if carers were better prepared to face changes in the patient as a person and in their relationship with the patient.

This study in a London health district differed from others (Wade and Langton-Hewer, 1985; Bamford *et al.*, 1986) in the high proportion of patients who were admitted directly to hospital without contacting their general practitioner. It was suggested that previous experience of the primary care service played some part in this, but the proximity of the district hospitals and the perception that help would be obtained more quickly there were probably the main factors. This has implications for the extent to which general practitioners were aware of what was happening, and for their ability to support the carer and to plan for support in the community. The advantages of home versus hospital continue to be debated, but there is little doubt that more of the patients in Greenwich could, with appropriate support, have been cared for initially at home (Wade and Langton-Hewer, 1985). The benefit of people being enabled to stay in their own family and social networks is probably underestimated.

Very few patients who arrive at casualty with a stroke fail to be admitted, although the provision of 24-hour district liaison nursing support, as is being tried in the Hackney health district of London (Bamford *et al.*, 1986), might provide the basis for more patients to be treated at home. Half the general practitioners in Greenwich indicated that they would like to care for more of their stroke patients at home, but current allocation of resources for treatment and rehabilitation militates against this.

The contribution of rehabilitation in hospital

Patients admitted to hospital appeared generally to be allocated to wards on the basis of bed availability rather than clinical criteria. However, the rehabilitation patients received was affected by the ward they were on. It follows that doctors in casualty influence the patient's future use of the services – a fact of which they should be aware. Since events in the first hours after the stroke appear to have such an important effect upon receipt of treatment and rehabilitation (see Chapters 3 and 4), it is important that doctors in casualty departments ensure appropriate assessments of patients, and subsequently that those assessments are available to and from those with the primary responsibility for care.

The effective distribution of resources for rehabilitation depends on a clearer idea of who will benefit, and on the availability of therapists, as well as on better organisation and communication in the hospital. In hospital, both patients and supporters identified a lack of involvement in rehabilitation, although this was the treatment which they most often felt could do some good. As in other studies, the effectiveness of rehabilitation was difficult to establish, but most patients were receiving two or three sessions every week. One approach to increasing effectiveness might be to recruit the willing carers into rehabilitation, providing them with skills with which they could increase their contribution to the patient's recovery. It should be possible for wards and departments to keep a record of contacts with carers, providing a form of internal audit on performance in this respect. There should, similarly, be a system within the hospital for recording and reporting the rehabilitation that stroke patients receive. The currently haphazard pattern of access to rehabilitation may not be apparent at consultant or ward level; its exposure should act as a tool for improving allocation of resources in each hospital – if there could be some consensus on which patients should be receiving which services.

It appeared that patients in the stroke unit made more functional improvement, and maintained their advantage over time. This result differs from that in the Edinburgh study (Garraway *et al.*, 1980*b*) and there is no consensus on the value of specialised units in the recovery phase (Royal College of Physicians, 1990). It does emphasise, though, the need to consider the implications of different approaches to assessment – measuring functional improvement, disability or change since before the stroke. The improved performance of stroke unit patients, which was particularly evident among those aged under 80, could have been due to a number of factors including greater use of rehabilitation, particularly occupational therapy, and the more useful involvement of carers by rehabilitation staff. The stroke unit was preferred for their patients by a majority of local general practitioners as the ward where greatest interest and initiative would be taken. The appropriate configuration of a stroke unit will differ in different areas, but the ingredients of a co-ordinated, specialist team dedicated to helping patients and their families could form the basis for care in many different environments – including the community outside hospital, where mobile stroke teams could offer some continuity and expertise in care.

Towards policies for care

The implications for practice in the various services and sectors have been presented tentatively because they are in so many cases quite general. There is a need for clearer explanation of prognoses and more timely information, continuity of interest and care, access to appropriate rehabilitation, training of patients and families to cope with new roles and risks, appreciation of the social and emotional problems caused by stroke, and acknowledgement of the central contribution of family carers. The breadth of these implications reflects the extensive changes wrought in the lives of patients and their families and the range of demands for adjusting to living with disablement – as regards housing, family relationships, leisure interests, domestic roles and personal identity, as well as the performance of physical activities. If services are going to improve the quality of life after stroke they must attend to the aspirations of the patients and their supporters, and to the limitations and restrictions in everyday life that are most important to them. They must also be guided by principles that maintain choice, including those of families who decide they cannot become the main carers.

The development of policies at various levels would provide a framework for the organisation and provision of services and for the supply of other requirements such as appropriate housing and leisure or day-care facilities. The existence of clear policies would also reflect some priority being given to stroke care. The current situation is one in which few such policies exist, due perhaps in part to a stark lack of evidence about which interventions or resources are most important or effective. The study in Greenwich identified some of the main gaps in provision as well as some of the preferences for care; it offers a basis for asserting that certain resources should be available less haphazardly, and this requires the formulation of discrete policies. These policies apply at various levels, from medical management and hospital organisation to issues of housing provision and employment.

The development of policies for *treatment* of stroke was central to a British consensus conference (King's Fund, 1988). This discussed the setting and monitoring of standards of care, which would be a major step forward – but the process will demand considerable goodwill as well as substantial insight from the diverse professional groups. There are obvious gaps in knowledge but also some obvious needs that can and should be met: for attention to social and family problems, for assessments of patients' emotional conditions, for information on the nature and causes of the stroke, for identification of difficulties in communication, and for providing families with skills and preparation for caring. A combination of monitoring by the hospital or general practitioner together with some consumer audit would show whether standards were being upheld. The same principles apply to policies for rehabilitation. In the current climate of uncertainties and caveats about the effectiveness of therapies it is not surprising that a systematic routine rarely exists. However, as part of any hospital stroke policy it will be essential to monitor who gets what – including rehabilitation. In a period of limited resources some system of triage (Garraway *et al.*, 1981*a*) is necessary; once adopted the system should be monitored and improved. These assessments of rehabilitation should include a consumer perspective, indicating whether rehabilitation relates to the preferences and aspirations of patients and carers. Their comments during the study reported here suggest that some rehabilitation activities are not meaningful to patients, as well as being judged ineffective as time passed after the stroke.

The objective of most current treatment after stroke is to improve physical performance and consequently quality of life. However, a consistent finding is the importance of context in translating physical disability into handicap. Treatment policies must address more directly the social, psychological, family and economic aspects of stroke, both to avoid some of the reasonably predictable sequelae for patients and their families, and to make use of opportunities to improve the situation. The role of carers and families must be foremost in these considerations; the assessment of carers' capacities and preferences should be a routine element in the management of stroke. The development of policies by *professional organisations* should have the effect of giving higher priority and more status to the care of stroke patients and their families.

Most workers have considered stroke patients as people for whom relatively little can be done. The reality of life after stroke appears in some ways directly to contradict this, insofar as there is a great deal that can be done and which is being done – but much of this activity demands leadership, co-ordination and continuing commitment. The complexity and multiplicity of agencies working to improve the situation after stroke leads to the needs for co-ordination of professional care and to ideas about 'key' workers, and to the need for integrated action by multi-professional teams. The health system in the United Kingdom is currently bounded by diverse barriers to a better integrated service, ranging from perceived threats to jobs and lack of time for meetings, to bureaucratic hurdles and a lack of positive incentives for professionals to work together. There is a lack of experience of working together and there are even difficulties in communication between professions. Trust and respect between professions are likely to emerge strongly only with experience of working together. However, communication and management may be assisted by the development of commonly understood and agreed methods of assessment, and by joint programmes of training. The need for training that is more sensitive and sympathetic to the needs of patients and their families has been mentioned for hospital nurses, rehabilitation staff and casualty doctors. A similar argument could be made for most of the professional groups involved in stroke care, acknowledging that there may also be a need for training in skills and understanding for working together. The efficacy of training for multi-professional teamwork is not well established and new schemes must be subject to evaluation before they become entrenched.

The development of stroke policies at *district* level picks up and extends the discussion of establishing effective mechanisms for community care through teams and key workers. The vital principle is the integration of the work of different professionals – integration between those in hospital and in the community, and between health, local government and voluntary services. A district stroke service will be made up from various models of organisation which will seek to maintain continuity and co-ordination between the different sources of help and support. These models will vary in different areas depending upon the existing levels of staff. However, in many areas the appropriate domiciliary rehabilitation services, particularly speech and physiotherapy, simply do not exist. The allocation of resources between hospital and community requires information about the places in which patients are cared for, their numbers and the resources they use. The implementation of a district stroke policy may also require the identification of a named individual (as foreseen in the King's Fund Statement 1988) who will be accountable for monitoring the service as well as for liaison with local government and other authorities. It has been evident for many years (Henwood, 1990) that the links between local government welfare services and health services are often tenuous and policies unco-ordinated, even though the health and welfare problems of patients and their families are strongly related. When the recommendations of the Griffiths Report (1988) on community care are implemented then responsibility for the design, co-ordination and purchase of non-health care services in the United Kingdom will pass to the local government social services departments.

These social services departments already play a vital role in facilitating care by families through the supportive and domestic services they make available. However, carers continued to want more help from social services than from other agencies and some needed reassurance that support would continue to flow. In Greenwich, sheltered housing was highly regarded by both patients and carers, but there were problems with other types of accommodation, from heating in rented accommodation to paying the rates in privately-owned homes. The prevalence of money worries and the incidence of financial loss caused by stroke, for both patients and carers, suggests that social services departments and social workers should participate more as sources of advice about and for other services, although more research into the effectiveness of such social work interventions is needed (Towle *et al.*, 1989). Most patients and carers need assistance in taking up the voluntary and statutory help available to them; the allowances, housing, holidays, respite services, support groups and employment opportunities available (about which social services are knowledgeable) are elements that may change the quality of life or handicaps suffered by patients and their families. As such, these services should be at the heart of a comprehensive policy for longer-term support after stroke.

The development of policies at a *national and governmental* level influences the extent to which change can be realised at other policy levels, through the priority and commitments given to resources for training, demonstration schemes, disability allowances, day-care centres and health or other services. The Griffiths Report (1988) specifies such objectives for government policy in the United Kingdom in terms of establishing a relationship between resources and policy that clarifies what it is the community care services are trying to achieve. It emphasises the need for flexibility and integration of services, with national policy providing the framework within which initiatives, innovation and commitment at the local level can flourish. While acknowledging the need to ensure adequate local performance, it is evident that the funds available are limited. However, the indications from trends in stroke incidence, against the background of an ageing population, are that the numbers of people with stroke are unlikely to fall. Although national policies in the last decade have been rephrased with explicit, rather than implicit, interaction between services and informal support networks, it is also clear that there may be changes in the cornerstone of national policy for care in the community – that is the capacity and preparedness of family carers, mainly women, to provide continuing care. Such changes may be difficult for national policies to control.

Many of the carers in the Greenwich study, particularly those of speech-impaired patients and the wives of patients, were suffering physically, socially and emotionally. In general a high proportion of carers, particularly those living with the dependent person, cope essentially 'single-handedly' (OPCS, 1988); once they have taken on the caring responsibilities they become isolated from friends and the help of services or other members of the family. In many ways the carers in Greenwich were disabled and handicapped by the stroke. There is a growing acknowledgement that becoming a carer often impoverishes that person's life. This, together with various demographic trends such as greater geographical mobility, divorce, lower birthrates and the increasing employment commitments of women, leads to 'considerable uncertainty' as to whether society can continue to expect the same levels of family care that exist today (Finch, 1989).

Carers must have a choice about caring, but there is nevertheless a lot that can be done to enhance the contribution of families and other sources of help and to improve the quality of carers' lives. Apart from policy initiatives to increase the volume and acceptability of respite care, family support groups, financial support and appropriate housing, the key lies in the systematic involvement of staff from health and social services: to prepare families for the future; to make appropriate use of available resources; to help maintain family relationships; and to transfer skills in caring and rehabilitation. There is growing pressure for service development and evaluation which embraces the needs and preferences of different groups of patients and carers, and a foundation of principles and experience exists upon which to strengthen that development (Trigg *et al.*, 1990; Henwood, 1990; Royal College of Physicians, 1990). The essentials for improved services to stroke patients and their carers are not a mystery.

Professionals increasingly recognise the contribution of the family; they know the importance of emotional and social problems; and they understand how problems, expectations and priorities change over time, thus demanding continuing support and assessment. The challenge is to translate this awareness into action.

Measurement and scoring of variables

A study of the factors influencing the quality of life of survivors of stroke and their main carers requires assessments ranging from clinical indicators of severity of stroke to measurement of aspects of stress and strain caused by the illness. The characteristics and lives of patients and their supporters cannot easily be summarised. Features such as disability, emotional distress and social activity are so multifaceted that they demand investigation of many aspects. These specific elements are discussed in the appropriate chapters, but comparisons between people or over time are generally presented in terms of summary scores. These scores have been derived from analysis of several items on 'measuring instruments' drawn from a variety of sources. In searching for appropriate instruments it was intended that they should ask questions which were relatively easy to answer, so that the maximum proportion of patients, including those with speech impairments, could give useful responses. The aim was for scoring to be based directly upon the responses of the patients and their supporters rather than on ratings by the researcher. As far as possible the same instruments were used with both patients and supporters.

The principal measures, their derivation, items and scoring are presented here. Items 1–3 describe the tests and assessments of patients that were made by the researcher.

1. Clinical

(a) Hemianopia/visual inattention: two pen test (Isaacs and Marks, 1973)

The examiner* sits immediately opposite the patient and asks the patient to look at his forehead. Two pens of different colour are held up simul-

---

* Throughout the Appendix, for reasons of clarity the examiner/researcher is assumed to be male and the patient is assumed to be female.

taneously about 30 cm in front of the patient and about 30 cm apart. The patient is asked what she sees. If only one of the pens can be seen their positions are interchanged before the patient's eyes and the question repeated. Patients with gross neglect report seeing only the pen on the unaffected side. Patients with hemianopia move their head towards the hemianopic side in order to bring the object into the unaffected visual field.

No attempt was made to distinguish hemianopia from inattention, so patients were rated as either normal or with neglect on the left or right side.

(b) Proprioception

The wrist of the affected arm is held by the examiner between his thumb and forefinger. The patient's hand is raised and lowered and then, with her eyes closed or covered, the patient is asked to indicate whether the hand is up or down. This is repeated several times with the hand both raised and lowered. After this the second finger of the affected hand is held in the middle between the examiner's thumb and forefinger. The distal and middle phalanges are raised and lowered and the patient, with her eyes closed or covered, is asked to indicate whether the finger is up or down. This is repeated several times with the finger both up and down.

The patient is assessed as having no loss of spatial sense, as having loss in the finger or a grosser loss in the wrist.

(c) Sensation: loss of superficial sensation in hand

The back of the patient's unaffected hand is stroked with the examiner's forefinger to check that the patient has sensation in this hand. The affected hand is then stroked with the same intensity while the patient's eyes are covered. The patient is asked to indicate whether (and where) she can feel the examiner's touch and if the sensation is the same as in the unaffected hand.

Where there is some sensation but less than in the unaffected hand the patient is rated as having reduced sensation.

(d) Sitting balance (modified after Wade et al., 1983)

The patient is asked if she is able to sit on the side of a bed with her feet off the floor and maintain balance. If she says that she can she is asked to demonstrate this, sitting unaided for 1 minute on the side of a firm bed.

Balance is rated as either normal or abnormal, the difference usually being readily apparent.

(e) Arm function (Prescott et al., 1982)

The patient is asked to lift the affected arm to shoulder height, and to push against the examiner's hand. Function is rated as:
- Complete paralysis: the patient is unable to move the arm and no flicker of muscular contraction is visible
- Severe weakness: the patient is able to move the affected arm but is unable to lift it to shoulder height and is unable to push against the examiner's hand
- Moderate weakness: the patient is able to lift the affected arm to shoulder height but is unable to push against the examiner's hand
- Slight weakness: the patient is able to lift the arm to shoulder height and is able to push the examiner's hand, but the affected limb is weaker than the unaffected one
- No weakness: no difference in the abilities of the affected and unaffected limb to push against the examiner's hand

These assessments were selected to cover important clinical predictors of physical recovery (Wade *et al.*, 1983). Another important factor was urinary incontinence.

2. Incontinence

Patients were rated on the following scale for both urine and faeces.
- Continent (includes managing a catheter/enema alone): scores 2
- Occasionally incontinent (includes needing help with an enema/catheter): scores 1
- Incontinent: scores 0

Patients rated as continent of both urine and faeces thus have a total score of 4. 'Occasional' is taken to mean incontinent of urine no more than once every 24 hours and incontinent of faeces no more than once every 48 hours.

3. Communication

(a) Comprehension (after Prescott et al., 1982)

The patient is asked to pick up a pen placed directly in front of her (as a prelude to writing her name). The patient's response is rated as:
- Communication easy: the patient is able to obey the verbal instruction

- Communication possible but difficult: the patient cannot follow the verbal command but is able to imitate the examiner carrying out the manoeuvre
- Communication not possible: the patient is totally unable to follow the instruction

(b) Expression (after Prescott et al., 1982)

Following the interview the patient's ability to express herself is rated as:
- Normal
- Impaired: the patient is able to convey meaning, but word formation is poor
- Absent: the patient is unable to convey any meaning (or simply cannot be understood)

4. Disability (Garrad and Bennett, 1971)

Garrad and Bennett (1971) described disability as 'limitation of performance in one or more activities which are generally accepted as essential basic components of daily living, such that inability to perform them necessitates dependence on another person' (p. 97). The content of their questionnaire was determined by definition of the essential activities of daily living, and can be divided into two parts: mobility and self-care. The individual questions and their scores are given in Table A.1 (p. 240).

(a) Mobility

(i) Transfer The question is designed to identify the patient who is unable to stand up vertically from a sitting position without help even though she may be able to slide from one chair to another or onto a commode.

(ii) Walking The criteria were abbreviated because of the limits of analysis; changing the distance from 100 yards to 50 yards makes it compatible with the Barthel score.

The question assumes a level surface and gives priority to walking outdoors. The patient is probed for level of performance and whether accompanied, unaccompanied or in a wheelchair. The patient's rating is defined as the highest level performance achieved with the least personal help – thus 10 yards unaccompanied rates a higher score than 50 yards accompanied. If performance is different in daylight and at night, daylight performance is recorded.

If the patient is unable to walk, questions are asked to establish whether she is independent for 50 yards in a wheelchair.

(iii) Stairs The patient may use any kind of walking aid or technique (including pauses) to walk (vertically) up or down stairs. If she crawls on all fours, or travels by sitting on successive stairs, this is recorded as 'other than walking'.

If the patient says she has no need to climb or descend stairs at home she is asked how she manages stairs in a friend's home, or the kerb if walking in the street.

(b) Self-care

Self-care is considered under five headings: feeding, dressing, washing, chiropody and toilet. The highest level of ability is that of a patient who is able to manage each activity completely without help from another, i.e. is completely independent. For each activity there are carefully defined grades, giving three categories of increasing severity of disability.

(i) Feeding
- Specially prepared food: the patient has, for example, food cut up, bread buttered (as for the hemiplegic or arthritic patient) or food arranged clockwise on the plate (as for a blind person) but needs no other help with feeding. Special containers, such as a non-spill beaker or beaker and tube as used by some neurological patients, may be required
- With assistance: the patient needs help from another person in addition to the above, e.g. needs the beaker held or steadied
- Must be fed: the severest grade of disability where the patient needs food put into her mouth

(ii) Dressing and undressing
- Help with fastenings: the patient can put on all her clothes but cannot manage the fastenings (buttons, shoe laces, etc.)
- Help other than fastenings: the patient needs help in putting the clothes on or arranging them
- Does not dress: the severest level of disability

(iii) Washing Washing is subdivided into grooming and bathing.
  The least severe grade of disability is that of the patient who needs help

only with combing hair, applying cosmetics, etc. – what might be termed the 'appearance' component of washing. In terms of daily living this could be restricted without too much disruption to the patient's life.

The patient who regularly needs help with washing any part of her body is more dependent and therefore more disabled. The severest level is that of the person who does not wash herself at all and is totally dependent on another person.

(iv) Chiropody This is often the first activity with which an elderly person needs help from someone else. If help is given by a member of the patient's household the situation is probably unchanged by the stroke. However, if the patient normally receives this care outside the house and is housebound as a result of the stroke, the lack of help may become a source of anxiety and discomfort. The question distinguishes between patients who either never, occasionally or always need help to cut their toenails.

(v) Use of the lavatory The rationale behind this question is that a patient is less disabled if she uses receptacles (e.g. commode) unaided than if she has to rely on another person to assist her in the use of the lavatory. Another person may have to empty the receptacles later, but the patient is not immediately dependent on another. The severest grade of disability is the patient who is only able to use receptacles with assistance at the time of use, e.g. bedfast patients who use a bed-pan. Some incontinent patients are catheterised; allowance is made for this to be coded. Some severely incapacitated bedfast patients are not given bed-pans, rather disposable bed linen is changed as necessary and the patient is cleaned. This situation is coded (rather inappropriately) as 'No care'.

Disability score and the Barthel score

Although the questionnaire developed by Garrad and Bennett (1971) is relatively comprehensive and sensitive for monitoring change, it was not designed for scoring on individual items or any statistical manipulation. Two changes were therefore made in the questions (on walking and washing) to make them comparable with the classification used to derive Barthel scores (Mahoney and Barthel, 1965). This had the benefit of permitting comparison with other studies that use Barthel scores. The questions, their coding and scoring are shown in Table A.1.

The total possible score, described in the text as the 'disability score', is 16 and is made up of two scores: mobility (score 0–8) and self-care (score

Table A.1. *Disability questions and scoring*

	Garrad & Bennett code	Disability Score (Based on Barthel)
Self-care		
Did/do you feed yourself:		
Without any help	1	2
With specially prepared food or containers	2	1
With assistance	3	
Not at all, must be fed	4	0
Did/do you dress yourself completely:		
Without any help	1	2
With help with fastenings	2	1
With help other than fastenings	3	
Does not dress	4	0
Did/do you wash your face, comb your hair, shave, clean your teeth:		
Yes, without help	1	1
No, help needed	2	0
Did/do you bath or wash yourself all over (with aids if used):		
Yes, bathing without help	3	1
Yes, standing wash without help	4	
No, need help with body washing	5	0
Did/do you use:		
Lavatory without help	1	2
Receptacles without assistance	2	
Lavatory with assistance	3	1
Receptacles with assistance	4	
Catheterised	5	0
No care	6	
Mobility		
Did/do you get out of bed:		
Unaided	1	Unaided for both bed and chair 3
With help	2	Unaided for one but other with help 2
Not at all (bedfast)	3	Both with help 0
		Bedfast (code 3)
If not bedfast		
Did/do you stand up from a chair:		
Unaided	4	
With help (chairfast)	5	

Did/do you walk outdoors in the
street (with a crutch or a stick, if
used):

Yes, outdoors: 440 yards	1	Independent for 50 yards or more	3	
50–440 yards	2	(1, 2, 3, 5 + A)		
10–50 yards	3	Able to walk (accompanied) > 50	2	
< 10 yards	4	yards (1, 2, 3, 5 + B)		
No, indoors: 50 yards	5			
10–50 yards	6			
< 10 yards	7			
Unable to walk	8	Unable to walk, but gets about in	1	
Not attempted	9	a wheelchair		

and:

Accompanied	A	
Unaccompanied	B	

If unable to walk (8)
Do you get about in a wheelchair:

Yes	1	Unable to walk, and unable to	0
No	2	get about in a wheelchair	

Did/do you walk up stairs or steps,
at home or elsewhere:

Yes: 5 stairs or more, unaccompanied	1	Walks up or mounts stairs unaccompanied (1, 2, 5)	2
1–4 stairs, unaccompanied	2	Goes up, but accompanied (3, 4)	1
5 stairs or more, accompanied	3	Unable, or does not mount stairs (6, 7, 8)	0
1–4 stairs, accompanied	4		
Mount stairs other than walking	5		
No, unable to mount stairs	6		
No need to mount stairs	7		
Not attempted	8		

0–8). When discussing life before the stroke a score of 15 or 16 is described
as 'no disability' or 'mild disability'. For life after the stroke the Barthel
score is generally used. This is derived by adding the disability score and
the continence score (see above), giving a range from 0 (completely
dependent) to 20 (independent). The Barthel score has been coded into
five ranges of disability: 0–4 (very severe); 5–9 (severe); 10–14 (moderate);
15–19 (mild) and 20 (normal). The mid-points of these ranges (2, 7, 12, 17
and 20) have been used to calculate average Barthel scores.

5. Orientation and memory (Isaacs and Walkey, 1963)

There are many relatively similar approaches to the global assessment of
orientation and memory, some of which are shorter and appear more
acceptable to patients (see Qureshi and Hodkinson, 1974). Here the
measure developed by Isaacs and Walkey is used, but omitting the item on

how long the patient had been in hospital so that the test was also appropriate for patients at home. Ultimately, this is the same test as used in the Edinburgh trial of stroke units (Prescott *et al.*, 1982). The patient is asked the following questions:

(*a*) What is the name of this place (address)?

(*b*) What day of the week is it today?

(*c*) What month is it?

(*d*) What year is it?

(*e*) What age are you? (an error of $\pm$ 1 year is allowed)

(*f*) In what year were you born?

(*g*) In what month is your birthday?

(*h*) Now, just a guess, what time is it? (an error of $\pm$ 1 hour is allowed)

One point is scored for each correct answer; the result is described in the text as the 'Walkey score'. In principle the lower the patient's Walkey score the greater the extent of loss of mental function, but it is not appropriate to be rigid about cut-off points. Patients can be classified into four groups on the basis of their score (see Prescott *et al.*, 1982), but here a distinction is generally drawn between those patients making three errors or more and the rest.

6. Housework activities (Holbrook and Skilbeck, 1983)

This measure has been abstracted from the factor analyses made by the authors of the Frenchay Activities Index, and the six items are presented and coded as in the original measure (which was developed for use with stroke patients). The examiner asks how often in the previous 3 months the patient:

(*a*) Prepared main meals: the patient needs to have played a substantial part in the organisation, preparation and cooking of the main meal. Making snacks is not sufficient

(*b*) Did the washing up: the patient must have done all the washing up after a meal, or shared the job equally with another (e.g. either washing, or wiping and putting away). Washing or wiping the occasional item is not sufficient

(*c*) Washed clothes: organisation or washing and drying of clothes, whether in a washing machine, by hand or at a laundrette

(*d*) Did light housework: dusting, vacuum cleaning one room

(*e*) Did heavy housework: all the housework including beds, floors, fires, etc.

(*f*) Did local shopping: the patient must have played a substantial role in organising and buying shopping, whether small or large amounts. Just pushing the trolley in the supermarket is not sufficient

Items (*a*) and (*b*) are scored as: never = 1; less than once a week = 2; once or twice a week = 3; most days = 4. Items (*c*) – (*f*) are scored as: never = 1; once or twice in 3 months = 2; three to twelve times in 3 months = 3; at least weekly = 4.

The total housework score is simply the result of adding the scores on each of the six items, giving a range from 6 to 24. For analysis the scores have been grouped into ranges as follows (the figure in brackets is the mid-point which has been used in calculating average scores): 6 (6); 7–10 (8.5); 11–14 (12.5); 15–18 (16.5); 19–22 (20.5); 23–24 (23.5).

7. Social activities

In the Frenchay Activities Index (Holbrook and Skilbeck, 1983) there is a single item that covers going out to clubs, church activities, cinema, theatre, drinking and to dinner with friends. Since the present study was specifically concerned with social aspects of stroke this item was expanded (during the pilot study) into a separate index. Patients and supporters were asked how often in the previous 3 months they had:

(*a*) Gone out to visit family or friends
(*b*) Gone to church
(*c*) Attended a social club
(*d*) Gone to the pub
(*e*) Gone on a day trip or outing
(*f*) Gone to a sports event, theatre or exhibition
(*g*) Had family or friends visit them at home

All items were coded and scored as: never = 1; once or twice in 3 months = 2; three to twelve times in 3 months = 3; at least once a week = 4.

The total social activities score is the sum of the scores on individual items, giving a range from 7 to 28. For analysis the scores have been coded into ranges as follows (the figure in brackets is the mid-point which has been used in calculating average scores): 7 (7); 8–11 (9.5); 12–15 (13.5); 16–19 (17.5); 20–23 (21.5); 24 or more (24).

The same questions were asked of the supporters about their social activities, except that the item on sports events, theatre and visits to museums or exhibitions was divided into two, so that sports events was one separate item and theatre, cinema and exhibitions was another. Scoring was the same as for the questions to patients, therefore giving a range of scores for supporters' social activities from 8 to 32. For analysis the scores were coded into the following ranges (mid-point in brackets): 8–11 (9.5); 12–15 (13.5); 16–19 (17.5); 20–23 (21.5); 24 or more (24).

It became apparent in early analyses that the social activities of patients consisted principally of visits to or from family and friends. The score on these two items from the social activities index is presented as a 'family contacts score', with a range from 2 to 8.

8. Subjective health (Hunt, McEwen and McKenna, 1984)

The patients' and supporters' subjective perceptions of their health were assessed using the Nottingham Health Profile. This investigates six aspects of health: emotional distress (EM), pain (P), energy (EN), sleep (SL), physical mobility (PM) and social isolation (SO). The supporters were asked to indicate whether each of 38 statements applied to them or not. The response set is, therefore, simply 'yes' or 'no'. The statements and the aspects of health to which they relate are shown in Table A.2.

This list was presented to supporters at each interview; most completed the responses themselves by hand, but for a minority the statements were read out and the interviewer checked off their responses on the questionnaire.

In the pilot study it became clear that the number of statements and their random ordering posed problems for patients. Ultimately only the statements relating to emotional distress and social isolation were presented to patients; and they were presented as two groups, each introduced with a cue to the theme of the statements (e.g. 'How do you feel in yourself?' or 'How do you feel with or towards other people?').

Positive responses to statements in the Nottingham Health Profile may be scored with different weights according to a system developed from an exercise in Thurstone scaling (McKenna *et al.*, 1981). However, very few of the people in that exercise were elderly, and it seems possible that the values that older people attach to different statements may be different from those of a younger population. For this reason, and because there are in practice many scores of 0, it was decided to score positive responses with equal weight, so that each 'yes' received a score of 1. The range of scores for the six aspects is thus: energy, 0–3; pain, 0–8; emotion, 0–9; physical mobility, 0–8; sleep, 0–5; social isolation, 0–5.

9. Stigma (Hyman, 1971)

Following the assessment of social isolation patients were asked whether they agreed or disagreed with three statements designed to assess feelings of being socially discredited. These statements are drawn from a previous study with stroke patients, although the wording of one item is slightly changed to accommodate English (as opposed to American) idiom. The statements are:

Table A.2. *Statements in the Nottingham Health Profile*

Statement	Code
I'm tired all the time	EN1
I have pain at night	P1
Things are getting me down	EM1
I have unbearable pain	P2
I take tablets to help me sleep	SL1
I've forgotten what it's like to enjoy myself	EM2
I'm feeling on edge	EM3
I find it painful to change position	P3
I feel lonely	SO1
I can only walk about indoors	PM1
I find it hard to bend	PM2
Everything is an effort	EN2
I'm waking up in the early hours of the morning	SL2
I'm unable to walk at all	PM3
I'm finding it hard to make contact with people	SO2
The days seem to drag	EM4
I have trouble getting up and down stairs or steps	PM4
I find it hard to reach for things	PM5
I'm in pain when I walk	P4
I lose my temper easily these days	EM5
I feel there is nobody I am close to	SO3
I lie awake for most of the night	SL3
I feel as if I'm losing control	EM6
I'm in pain when I'm standing	P5
I find it hard to dress myself	PM6
I soon run out of energy	EN3
I find it hard to stand for long (e.g. at the kitchen sink, waiting for a bus)	PM7
I'm in constant pain	P6
It takes me a long time to get to sleep	SL4
I feel I am a burden to people	SO4
Worry is keeping me awake at night	EM7
I feel that life is not worth living	EM8
I sleep badly at night	SL5
I'm finding it hard to get on with people	SO5
I need help to walk about outside (e.g. a walking aid or someone to support me)	PM8
I'm in pain when going up and down stairs or steps	P7
I wake up feeling depressed	EM9
I'm in pain when I'm sitting	P8

(a) I feel that other people are uncomfortable with me

(b) I feel other people treat me like an inferior person

(c) I feel other people would prefer to avoid me

Each 'yes' response was given a score of 1, producing a total score in the range 0–3.

10. Subjective stress

We used several approaches to assess the effects of the stroke on the supporters. They were asked about the burden caused by the stroke, about life satisfaction, about subjective health and, at all three interviews, about their assessment of stress in their everyday life. This last indicator asks supporters to what extent they agree with the following four statements:

(a) At the end of the day I am completely exhausted, mentally and physically

(b) There is a great amount of nervous strain associated with my daily activities

(c) My daily activities are extremely trying and stressful

(d) In general I am usually tense and nervous

Responses are invited and scored as: strongly agree = 4; agree = 3; disagree = 2; strongly disagree = 1. These scores are summed to give a total score, ranging from 4 (low stress) to 16 (high stress). These total scores have been coded into the following groups for analysis (The figure in brackets is the mid-point which has been used for calculating average scores): 4 (4); 5–6 (5.5); 7–8 (7.5); 9–10 (9.5); 11–12 (11.5); 13–14 (13.5); 15–16 (15.5).

11. Interaction (after Venters, 1981)

This measure of interaction was originally one part of an index of family functioning in chronic illness, and is used here to express some positive aspects of the relationship between the patient and supporter. The supporter was asked, at all three interviews, how frequently (never, some-times, often), he or she and the patient:

(a) Had an enjoyable conversation together

(b) Laughed about something together

(c) Felt close to one another

(d) Looked forward to doing something together

Clearly some of these experiences may be reduced by the direct, physical effects of the stroke. Therefore this index is described as a measure of 'interaction', rather than of, say, quality of relationship, as this reflects in practice what it is. The items are scored as: never = 0; sometimes = 1; often = 2. The total score thus has a range from 0 (low) to 8 (high).

12. Irritation (after Gilleard et al., 1984)

From the six items in the interaction scale used by the psychogeriatric day care research project in Edinburgh, four negative items – anger, interference, tension and upsets – were selected to reflect some of the negative aspects of the relationship between the supporter and patient. Supporters were asked, at each interview, how frequently they:

(*a*) Felt cross or angry with patient
(*b*) Felt that the patient was interfering too much (in their life, family, household)
(*c*) Felt tension in their relationship with the patient
(*d*) Had upsetting disagreements with the patient

The items are scored as: never = 0; sometimes = 1; often = 2. The total score thus has a range from 0 to 8, a higher score indicating more irritation.

13. Patient's mood

Discussions of changes in the patient's 'personality' or 'mood' following stroke are commonplace, but there has never been an attempt systematically to document these changes in everyday, as opposed to psychotic, behaviour. Other studies of changes in the mood of patients with senile dementia (Greene *et al.*, 1982; Levin *et al.*, 1983) and with heart disease (Croog and Levine, 1977) were used to identify items, and these were investigated in the pilot study. In the main study supporters were asked at all three interviews how often the patient was:

(*a*) Warm and affectionate towards you
(*b*) Complaining and critical
(*c*) Aggressive or bad-tempered
(*d*) Cheerful
(*e*) Demanding attention
(*f*) Alert and interested
(*g*) Irritable and easily upset
(*h*) Appreciative of things you did
(*i*) Depressed

The responses were scored as: never = 0; sometimes = 1; often = 2. The

Appendix

nine items were placed into two groups for scoring: positive (items (*a*), (*d*), (*f*) and (*h*)) and negative (items (*b*), (*c*), (*e*), (*g*) and (*i*)). The total score for positive mood is from 0 to 8, and for negative mood from 0 to 10.

14. Change scores

Changes in the scores for disability, housework, social activities, subjective health, stress, interaction, irritation and mood were also analysed. In all cases the actual score, not the coded range, has been used to calculate the change score.

References

Abramson, L. Y., Seligman, M. E. and Teasdale, J. D. (1978) Learned helplessness in humans: critique and reformulation. *J. Abnorm. Psychol.* **87**, 49–74.

Abu-Zeid, H. A. H., Won Choi, N., Hsu, P.-H. and Maini, K. K. (1978) Prognostic factors in the survival of 1484 stroke cases observed for 30 to 48 months. I. Diagnostic types and descriptive variables. *Arch. Neurol.* **35**, 121–5.

Adams, G. F. (1974) Cerebrovascular disability and the ageing brain. Edinburgh: Churchill Livingstone.

Adams, G. F. and Merrett, J. D. (1961) Prognosis and survival in the aftermath of hemiplegia. *Br. Med. J.* **i**, 309–14.

Aho, K., Harmsen, P., Hatano, S. *et al.* (1980) Cerebrovascular disease in the community: results of a WHO collaborative study. *Bull. WHO* **58**(1), 113–30.

Allen, I., Wicks, M., Finch, J. and Leat, D. (1987) *Informal care tomorrow*. London: Policy Studies Institute.

Alonzo, A. A. (1980) Acute illness behaviour: a conceptual exploration and specification. *Soc. Sci. Med.* **14A**, 515–26.

Anderson, R. M. (1987) The unremitting burden on carers. *Br. Med. J.* **294**, 73–4.

Anderson, R. M. (1988) The quality of life of stroke patients and their carers. In: *Living with chronic illness*, ed. R. Anderson and M. Bury, pp. 14–42. London: Unwin Hyman.

Anderson, T. P., Baldridge, M. and Ettinger, M. G. (1979) Quality of care for completed stroke without rehabilitation: evaluation by assessing patient outcomes. *Arch. Phys. Med. Rehabil.* **60**, 103–7.

Andrews, F. M. and Withey, S. B. (1976) *Social indicators of well being*. New York: Plenum Press.

Andrews, K. and Stewart, J. (1979) Stroke recovery: he can but does he? *Rheumatol. Rehabil.* **18**(1), 43–8.

Arber, S., Gilbert, N. and Evandrou, M. (1988) Gender, household composition and receipt of domiciliary services by the elderly disabled. *J. Soc. Policy* **17**(2), 153–75.

Artes, R. and Hoops, R. (1976) Problems of aphasic and non-aphasic stroke patients as identified and evaluated by patients' wives. In: *Recovery in aphasics*, ed. Y. Lebrun and R. Hoops. Amsterdam: Swets and Zeitlinger.

Askham J. (1982) Professionals criteria for accepting people as patients. *Soc. Sci. Med.* **16**, 2083–9.

Baker, R. N., Schwartz, W. S. and Ramseyer, J. C. (1968) Prognosis among survivors of ischemic stroke. *Neurology* **18**, 933–41.

Bamford, J. M., Sandercock, P. A. G., Warlow, C. P. and Gray, J. M. (1986) Why are patients with acute stroke admitted to hospital? *Br. Med. J.* **292**, 1369–72.

Bamford, J., Sandercock, P., Dennis, M., Burn, J. and Warlow, C. (1990) A prospective study of acute cerebrovascular disease in the community: the Oxfordshire Community Stroke Project 1981–86. II. Incidence, case fatality rates, and overall outcome at one year of cerebral infarction, primary intracerebral and subarachnoid haemorrhage. *J. Neurol. Neurosurg. Psychiatry* **53**, 16–22.

Belcher, S. A., Clowers, M. R. and Cabanayan, A. C. (1978) Independent living rehabilitation needs of postdischarge stroke persons: a pilot study. *Arch. Phys. Med. Rehabil.* **59**, 404–9.

Blaxter, M. (1976) *The meaning of disability*. London: Heinemann.

Blower, P. and Ali, S. (1979) A stroke unit in a district general hospital: the Greenwich experience. *Br. Med. J.* **ii**, 644–6.

Brocklehurst, J. C., Andrews, K., Morris, P. E. *et al.* (1978a) *Medical, social and psychological aspects of stroke*. Final Report to the Department of Health and Social Security.

Brocklehurst, J. C., Andrews, K., Morris, P. *et al.* (1978b) Why admit stroke patients to hospital? *Age Ageing* **7**, 100–8.

Brocklehurst, J. C., Andrews, K., Richards, B. and Laycock, P. J. (1978c) How much physical therapy for patients with stroke? *Br. Med. J.* **i**, 1307–10.

Brocklehurst, J. C., Morris, P., Andrews, K. *et al.* (1981) Social effects of stroke. *Soc. Sci. Med.* **15A**, 35–9.

Brust, J. C. M., Shafer, S. Q., Richter, R. W. *et al.* (1976) Aphasia in acute stroke. *Stroke* **7**, 167–74.

Bury, M. R. (1979) Disablement in society: towards an integrated perspective. *Int. J. Rehabil. Res.* **2**, 33–40.

Bury, M. R. (1987) The ICIDH: a review of research and prospects. *Int. Disability Stud.* **9**, 118–28.

Carstairs, V. (1976) Stroke: resource consumption and the cost to the community. In: *Stroke*, ed. F..J. Gillingham, C. Mawdsley and A. E. Williams. Edinburgh: Churchill Livingstone.

Cartwright, A. (1964) *Human relations and hospital care*. London: Routledge & Kegan Paul.

Cartwright, A. (1967) *Patients and their doctors*. London: Routledge & Kegan Paul.

Cartwright, A. and Anderson, R. (1981) *General practice revisited*. London: Tavistock.

Cartwright, A. and Henderson G. (1986) *More trouble with feet: a survey of foot problems and chiripody needs of the elderly*. London: HMSO.

Cartwright, A. and Smith, C. (1988) *Elderly people, their medicines and their doctors*. London: Routledge.

Chin, P. L., Angunawela, R., Mitchell, D. and Horne, J. (1980) Stroke register in Carlisle: a preliminary report. In: *Clinical neuroepidemiology*, ed. A. C. Rose, pp. 131–43. Tunbridge Wells: Pitman Medical.

Christie, D. (1982) Aftermath of stroke: an epidemiological study in Melbourne, Australia. *J. Epidemiol. Community Health* **36**, 123–6.

Christie, D. and Lawrence, L. (1978) Patients and hospitals: a study of the attitudes of stroke patients. *Soc. Sci. Med.* **12**, 49–51.

Coughlan, A. K. and Humphrey, M. (1982) Presenile stroke: long term outcome for patients and their families. *Rheumatol. Rehabil.* **21**, 115–22.

Croog, S. H. and Levine, S. (1977) *The heart patient recovers: social and psychological factors*. New York: Human Sciences Press.

Currie, C. T. (1986) Urinary incontinence after stroke. *Br. Med. J.* **293**, 1322–3 and 1524.

D'Afflitti, J. G. and Weitz, G. W. (1977) Rehabilitating the stroke patient through patient–family groups. In: *Coping with physical illness*, ed. R. H. Moos. New York: Plenum Press.

David, R., Enderby, P. and Bainton, D. (1982) Treatment of acquired aphasia: speech therapists and volunteers compared. *J. Neurol. Neurosurg. Psychiatry* **45**, 957–61.

Davies, P., Bamford, J. and Warlow, C. (1989) Remedial therapy and functional recovery in a total population of first-stroke patients. *Int. J. Disability Stud.* **11**(1), 40–4.

Department of Health and Social Security (1985) *Health and personal social services statistics for England: 1985 Edition*. London, HMSO.

Dzau, R. E. and Boehme, A. R. (1978) Stroke rehabilitation: a family-team education program. *Arch. Phys. Med. Rehabil.* **59**, 236–9.

Ebrahim, S., Barer, D. and Nouri, F. (1986) Use of the Nottingham Health Profile with patients after a stroke. *J. Epidemiol. Community Health* **40**, 166–9.

Engel, G. I. (1977) The need for a new medical model: a challenge for biomedicine. *Science* **196**, 129–36.

Evans, J. G. (1979) The epidemiology of stroke. *Age Ageing* [Supp] 50–6.

Feibel, J. H. and Springer, C. J. (1982) Depression and failure to resume social activities after stroke. *Arch. Phys. Med. Rehabil.* **63**, 276–8.

Feigenson, J. S., Gitlow, H. S. and Greenberg, S. D. (1979) The disability oriented rehabilitation unit: a major factor influencing stroke outcome. *Stroke* **10**, 5–8.

Feigenson, J. S., McDowell, F. H., Meese, P. *et al.* (1977a) Factors influencing outcome and length of stay in a stroke rehabilitation unit. I. Analysis of 248 unscreened patients: medical and functional prognostic indicators. *Stroke* **8**, 651–6.

Feigenson, J. S., McCarthy, M. L., Greenberg, S. D. and Feigenson, W. D. (1977b) Factors influencing outcome and length of stay in a stroke rehabilitation unit. II. Comparison of 318 screened and 248 unscreened patients. *Stroke* **8**, 657–62.

Feldman, D. J., Lee, P. R., Unterecker, J. *et al.* (1962) A comparison of functionally orientated medical care and formal rehabilitation in the management of patients with hemiplegia due to cerebrovascular disease. *J. Chronic Dis.* **15**, 297–310.

Field, D., Cordle, C. J. and Bowman, G. S. (1983) Coping with 'stroke at home'. *Int. Rehabil. Med.* **5**, 96–100.

Finch, J. (1989) *Family obligations and social change.* Cambridge: Polity Press.

Finch, J. and Groves, D. (1983) A labour of love: women, work and caring. London: Routledge & Kegan Paul.

Folstein, M. F., Maiberger, R. and McHugh, P. R. (1977) Mood disorder as a specific complication of stroke. *J. Neurol. Neurosurg. Psychiatry* **40**, 1018–20.

Ford, A. B. and Katz, S. (1966) Prognosis after strokes. I. A critical review. *Medicine* **45**, 223–36.

Forer, S. K. and Miller, L. S. (1980) Rehabilitation outcome: comparative analysis of different patient types. *Arch. Phys. Med. Rehabil.* **61**, 359–65.

Fullerton, K. J., McSherry, D. and Stout, R. W. (1986) Albert's test: a neglected test of perceptual neglect. *Lancet* **i**, 430–2.

Garrad, J. and Bennett, A. E. (1971) A validated interview schedule for use in population surveys of chronic disease and disability. *Br. J. Prev. Soc. Med.* **25** 97–104.

Garraway, W. M., Akhtar, A. J., Hockey, L. and Prescott, R. J. (1980*a*) Management of acute stroke in the elderly: follow-up of a controlled trial. *Br. Med. J.* **281**, 827–9.

Garraway, W. M., Akhtar, A. J., Prescott, R. J. and Hockey, L. (1980*b*) Management of acute stroke in the elderly: preliminary results of a controlled trial. *Br. Med. J.* **280**, 1040–3.

Garraway, W. M., Akhtar, A. J., Smith, D. L. and Smith, M. E. (1981*a*) The triage of stroke rehabilitation. *J. Epidemiol. Community Health* **35**, 39–44.

Garraway, W. M., Walton, M. S., Akhtar, A. J. and Prescott, R. J. (1981*b*). The use of health and social services in the management of stroke in the community: results from a controlled trial. *Age Ageing* **10**, 95–104.

Gilleard, C. J., Gilleard, E., Gledhill, K. and Whittick, J. (1984) Care for the elderly mentally infirm at home: a survey of the supporters. *J. Epidemiol. Community Health* **38**, 319–25.

Goldberg, D. (1985) Identifying psychiatric illness among general medical patients. *Br. Med. J.* **291**, 161–2.

Granger, C. V., Dewis, L. S., Peters, N. C. *et al.* (1979) Stroke rehabilitation: analysis of repeated Barthel index measures. *Arch. Phys. Med. Rehabil.* **60**, 14–17.

Greene, J. G., Smith, R., Gardiner, M. and Timbury, G. C. (1982) Measuring behavioural disturbance of elderly demented patients in the community and its effects on relatives: a factor analytic study. *Age Ageing* **11**, 121–6.

Griffiths, R. (1988) *Community care: agenda for action.* A report to the Secretary of State for Social Services. London: HMSO.

Haberman, S., Capildeo, R. and Rose, F. C. (1981) Sex differences in the incidence of cerebrovascular disease. *J. Epidemiol. Community Health* **35**, 45–50.

Hasler, J. C. (1985) The very stuff of general practice. *J. R. Coll. Gen. Pract.* **35**, 121–7.

Henderson, S., Byrne, D. G., Duncan-Jones, P. *et al.* (1980) Social relationships, adversity and neurosis: a study of associations in a general population sample. *Br. J. Psychiatry* **136**, 574–83.

Henley, S., Petit, S., Todd-Pokropek, A. and Tupper, A. (1985) Who goes home? Predictive factors in stroke recovery. *J. Neurol. Neurosurg. Psychiatry* **48**, 1–6.

Henwood, M. (1990) *Community care and elderly people*. London: Family Policy Studies Centre.

Herman, B., Schulte, B. P. M., Van Luijk, J. H. *et al.* (1980) Epidemiology of stroke in Tilburg, The Netherlands. The population-based stroke incidence register. I. Introduction and preliminary results. *Stroke* **11**, 162–5.

Hewer, R. L. (1976) Stroke rehabilitation. In: *Stroke*, ed, F. Gillingham *et al.* Edinburgh: Churchill Livingstone.

Holbrook, M. (1982) Stroke: social and emotional outcome. *J. R. Coll Physicians Lond.* **16** (2), 100–4.

Holbrook, M. and Skilbeck, C. E. (1983) An activities index for use with stroke patients. *Age Ageing* **12**, 166–70.

House, A. (1987) Depression after stroke. *Br. Med. J.* **294**, 76–8.

House, A., Dennis, M., Hawton, K. and Warlow, C. (1989) Methods of identifying mood disorders in stroke patients: experience in the Oxfordshire Community Stroke Project. *Age Ageing* **18**, 371–9.

Hunt, S. M., McEwen, J. M. and McKenna, S. P. (1984) Perceived health: age and sex comparisons in a community. *J. Epidemiol. Community Health* **38**, 156–60.

Hurwitz, L. J. and Adams, G. F. (1972) Rehabilitation of hemiplegia: indices of assessment and prognosis. *Br. Med. J.* **i**, 94–8.

Hyman, M. D. (1971) The stigma of stroke. *Geriatrics* [May], 132–41.

Hyman, M. D. (1972) Social isolation and performance in rehabilitation. *J. Chronic Dis.* **25**, 85–97.

Illsley, R. (1980) *Profession or public health*? London: Nuffield Provincial Hospitals Trust.

Isaacs, B. (1977) Five years' experience of a stroke unit. *Health Bull.* **35**, 94–8.

Isaacs, B. and Marks, R. (1973) Determinants of outcome of stroke rehabilitation. *Age Ageing* **2**, 139–49.

Isaacs, B. and Walkey, F. A. (1963) The assessment of the mental state of elderly hospital patients using a simple questionnaire. *Am. J. Psychiatry* **120**, 173–4.

Isaacs, B., Neville, Y. and Rushford I. (1976) The stricken: the social consequences of stroke. *Age Ageing* **5**, 188–92.

Jones, D. A. and Vetter, N. J. (1985) Formal and informal support received by carers of elderly dependents. *Br. Med. J.* **291**, 643–5.

King's Fund (1988) Consensus conference: the treatment of stroke. *Br. Med. J.* **297**, 126–8.

Kinsella, G. J. and Duffy, F. D. (1979) Psychosocial readjustment in the spouses of aphasic patients: a comparative survey of 79 subjects. *Scand. J. Rehabil. Med.* **11**, 129–32.

Labi, M., Phillips, T. F. and Gresham, G. E. (1980) Psychosocial disability in physically restored long-term stroke survivors. *Arch. Phys. Med. Rehabil.* **61**, 561–5.

Lancet (editorial) (1981) The stroke patient in hospital. *Lancet* **i**, 927–8.

Lawrence, L. and Christie, D. (1979) Quality of life after stroke: a three year follow-up. *Age Ageing* **8**, 167–72.

Legh-Smith, J., Wade, D. T. and Langton-Hewer, R. (1986) Services for stroke patients one year after stroke. *J. Epidemiol. Community Health* **40**, 161–5.

Lehmann, J. F., DeLateur, B. J., Fowler, R. S. *et al.* (1975a), Stroke: does rehabilitation affect outcome? *Arch. Phys. Med. Rehabil.* **56**, 375–82.

Lehmann, J. F., DeLateur, B. L., Fowler, R. S. *et al.* (1975b) Stroke rehabilitation: outcome and prediction. *Arch. Phys. Med. Rehabil.* **56**, 383–9.

Levin, E., Sinclair, I. A. C. and Gorbach, P. (1983) *The supporters of elderly persons at home*. Report to Department of Health and Social Security.

Levine, J. and Zigler, E. (1975) Denial and self-image in stroke, lung cancer and heart disease patients. *J. Consult. Clin. Psychiatry* **43**, 751–7.

Lincoln, N. B., McGuirk, E., Mulley, G. P. *et al.* (1984) Effectiveness of speech therapy for aphasic stroke patients: a randomised controlled trial. *Lancet* **i**, 1197–200.

Litman, T. J. (1962) Self-conception and physical rehabilitation. In: *Human behaviour and social processes*, ed. A. M. Rose, pp. 550–74. Boston: Houghton Miffin.

Locker, D. (1983) *Disability and disadvantage: the consequences of chronic illness*. London: Tavistock.

London Health Planning Consortium (1981) *Primary health care in Inner London* (the Acheson Report). London: LHPC.

McKenna, S. P., Hunt, S. M. and McEwen, J. (1981) Weighting the seriousness of perceived health problems usuing Thurstone's method of paired comparisons. *Int. J. Epidemiol.* **10**, 93–7.

Mackay, A. and Nias, B. C. (1979) Strokes in the young and middle-aged: consequences to the family and to society. *J. R. Coll. Physician's Lond.* **13**, 106–12.

Mahoney, F. I. and Barthel, D. W. (1965) Functional evaluations: the Barthel index. *Maryland State Med. J.* **14**, 61–5.

Malone, R. L. Olacek, P. M. and Malone, M. S. (1979) Attitudes expressed by families of aphasics. *Br. J. Disord. Commun.* **5**, 174–9.

Marquardsen, J. (1969) The natural history of acute cerebrovascular disease: a retrospective study of 769 patients. *Acta Neurol. Scand.* **45** [Supple 38].

Mayou, R. (1986) The psychiatric and social consequences of coronary artery surgery. *J. Psychosom. Res.* **30**, 255–71.

Morrissey, M., Mitchell, M. and Alaszewski, A. (1981) *The home care of elderly stroke patients*. University of Hull: Institute for Health Studies.

Mulhall, D. J. (1978) Dysphasic stroke patients and the influence of their relatives. *Br. J. Disord. Commun.* **13**, 127–34.

Mulley, G. (1981) Stroke rehabilitation: what are we all doing? In: *Health care of the elderly*, ed. T. Arie. London: Croom Helm.

Mulley, G. and Arie, T. (1978) Treating stroke: home or hospital. *Br. Med. J.* **ii**, 1321–2.

Murray, S. K., Garraway, W. M., Akhtar, A. J. and Prescott, R. J. (1982) Communication between home and hospital in the management of acute stroke in the elderly: results from a controlled trial. *Health Bull.* **40**, 214–19.

Mykyta, L. J., Bowling, J. H., Nelson, D. A. and Lloyd, E. J. (1976) Caring for relatives of stroke patients. *Age Ageing* 5, 87–90.

New, P. K.-M., Ruscio, A. T., Priest, R. P., Petritsi, D. and George, L. A. (1968) The support structure of heart and stroke patients. *Soc. Sci. Med.* 2, 185–200.

Newman, S. (1984) The social and emotional consequences of head injury and stroke. *Int. Rev. Appl. Psychol.* 33, 427–55.

Norris, J. W. and Hachinski, V. C. (1982) Misdiagnosis of stroke. *Lancet* i, 328–31.

Office of Population Censuses and Surveys (1982) *General household survey 1980.* London: HMSO.

Office of Population Censuses and Surveys (1985) Deaths: selected causes and sex. *Pop. Trends* 41, 50–1.

Office of Population Censuses and surveys (1988) *General household survey 1985: Informal carers.* London: HMSO.

Oxbury, J. K., Greenhall, R. C. D. and Grainger, K. M. R. (1975) Predicting the outcome of stroke: acute stage after cerebral infarction. *Br. Med. J.* iii, 125–7.

Oxfordshire Community Stroke Project (1983) Incidence of stroke in Oxford-shire: first year's experience of a community stroke register. *Br. Med. J.* 287, 713–17.

Peacock, P. B., Riley, C. P., Lampton, D. *et al.* (1972) The Birmingham stroke epidemiology and rehabilitation study. In: *Trends in epidemiology: application to health services research and training*, ed. G. T. Stewart. Springfield, Illinois: C. C. Thomas.

Pearlin, L. I. and Schooler, C. (1978) The structure of coping. *J. Health Soc. Behav.* 19, 2–21.

Prescott, R. J., Garraway, W. M. and Akhtar, A. J. (1982) Predicting functional outcome following acute stroke using a standard clinical examination. *Stroke* 13, 641–7.

Qureshi, K. N. and Hodkinson, H. M. (1974) Evaluation of a ten-question mental test in the institutionalised elderly. *Age Ageing* 3, 152–7.

Radic, A., Finn, A., Aran, R. and Dean, G. (1977) Incidence of strokes in Dublin. *Irish Med. J.* 70, 591–6.

Robertson, E. K. and Suinn, R. M. (1968) The determination of rate of progress of stroke patients through empathy measures of patient and family. *J. Psychosom. Res.* 12, 189–91.

Robinson, R. G. and Price, T. R. (1982) Post-stroke depressive disorders: a follow-up study of 103 patients. *Stroke* 13, 635–41.

Robinson, R. G., Bolduc, P. L., Kubos, K. L., Starr, L. B. and Price, T. R. (1985) Social functioning assessment in stroke patients. *Arch. Phys. Med. Rehabil.* 66, 496–500.

Royal College of General Practitioners, OPCS and DHSS (1982) *Morbidity statistics from general practice 1970–71: socio-economic analyses.* Studies on Medical and Population Subjects No. 46. London: HMSO.

Royal College of Physicians (1986) Physical disability in 1986 and beyond: a report of the Royal College of Physicians. *J. R. Coll. Physicians Lond.* 20, 160–94.

Royal College of Physicians (1990) Stroke: towards better management – summary and recommendations. *J. R. Coll. Physicians Lond.* **24**, 15–17.

Sacco, R. L., Wolf, P. A., Kannel, W. B. and McNamara, P. M. (1982) Survival and recurrence following stroke: the Framingham study. *Stroke* **13**, 290–5.

Sanford, J. R. A. (1975) Tolerance of debility in elderly dependants by supporters at home: its significance for hospital practice. *Br. Med. J.* **iii**, 471–3.

Seifert, K. H. (1979). The attitudes of working people towards disabled persons, especially in regard to vocational rehabilitation (research abstract). *Int. J. Rehabil. Res* **2**, 79–80.

Shanas, E. (1979) The family as a social support system in old age. *Gerontologist* **19**, 169–74.

Sheikh, K., Smith, D. S., Meade, T. W. *et al.* (1979) Repeatability and validity of a modified activities of daily living (ADL) index in studies of chronic disability. *Int. Rehabil. Med.* **1**, 51–8.

Sheikh, K., Brennan, P. J., Meade, T. W., Smith, D. S. and Goldenberg, E. (1983) Predictors of mortality and disability in stroke. *J. Epidemiol. Community Health* **37**, 70–4.

Smith, D. S., Goldenberg, E., Ashburn, A. *et al.*, (1981) Remedial therapy after stroke: a randomised controlled trial. *Br. Med. J.* **282**, 517–20.

Smith, M., Walton, M. S. and Garraway, W. M. (1981) The use of aids and adaptations in a study of stroke rehabilitation. *Health Bull.* **39**, 98–106.

Smith, R. T. (1979) Rehabilitation of the disabled: the role of social networks in the recovery process. *Int. Rehabil. Med.* **1**, 63–72.

Social Services Inspectorate (1987) *From home help to home care: an analysis of policy, resourcing and service management.* London: SSI Department of Health and Social Security.

Stevens, R. S. and Ambler, N. R. (1982) The incidence and survival of stroke patients in a defined community. *Age Ageing* **11**, 266–74.

Sussman, M. (ed.) (1965) *Sociology and rehabilitation.* Washington, DC: American Sociological Association.

Towle, D., Lincoln, N. B. and Mayfield, L. M. (1989) Service provision and functional independence in depressed stroke patients, and the effect of social work intervention on these. *J. Neurol. Neurosurg. Psychiatry* **52**, 519–22.

Twigg, J., Atkin, K. and Perring, C. (1990) *Carers and services: a review of research.* London: HMSO

Twining, T. C. and Chapman, J. R. (1980) Management of acute stroke in the elderly. *Br. Med. J.* **281**, 1142.

Venters, M. (1981) Familial coping with chronic and severe childhood illness: the case of cystic fibrosis. *Soc. Sci. Med.* **15A**, 289–97.

Vetter. N. J. (1980) Home or hospital for the stroke patient? *Lancet* **ii**, 1254.

Wade, D. T. (1984) An assessment of domiciliary care for acute stroke. MD Thesis, University of Cambridge.

Wade, D. T. and Langton-Hewer, R. (1985) Hospital admission for acute stroke: who, for how long, and to what effect? *J. Epidemiol. Community Health* **39**, 347–52.

Wade, D. T. and Langton-Hewer, R. (1987*a*) Functional abilities after stroke: measurement, natural history and prognosis. *J. Neurol. Neurosurg. Psychiatry* **50**, 177–82.

Wade, D. T. and Langton-Hewer, R. (1987*b*) Epidemiology of some neurological diseases. *Int. Rehabil. Med.* **8**, 129–37.

Wade, D. T., Skilbeck, C. E. and Langton-Hewer, R. (1983) Predicting Barthel ADL Score at 6 months after an acute stroke. *Arch. Phys. Med. Rehabil.* **64**, 24–8.

Wade, D. T., Skilbeck, C. E., Langton-Hewer, R. L. and Wood, V. A. (1984). Therapy after stroke: amounts, determinants and effects. *Int. Rehabil. Med.* **6**(3), 105–10.

Wade, D. T., Langton-Hewer, R., Skilbeck, C. E., Bainton, D. and Burns-Cox, C. (1985*a*) Controlled trial of a home-care service for acute stroke patients. *Lancet* **i**, 323–6.

Wade, D. T., Legh-Smith, J. and Langton-Hewer, R. (1985*b*) Social activities after stroke: measurement and natural history using the Frenchay Activities Index. *Int. Rehabil. Med* **7**, 176–81.

Wade, D. T., Legh-Smith, J. and Langton-Hewer, R. (1986*a*) Effects of living with and looking after survivors of stroke. *Br. Med. J.* **293**, 418–20.

Wade, D. T., Langton-Hewer, R., David, R. M. and Enderby, P. M. (1986*b*) Aphasia after stroke: natural history and associated deficits. *J. Neurol. Neurosurg. Psychiatry* **49**, 11–16.

Wade, D. T., Legh-Smith, J. and Langton-Hewer, R. (1987) Depressed mood after stroke. *Br. J. Psychiatry* **151**, 200–5.

Warlow, C., Wade, D., Sandercock, P. *et al.*, (1987) *Strokes*. Lancaster: MTP Press.

Weddell, J. M. and Beresford, S. A. A. (1979) *Planning for stroke patients*. London: HMSO.

Wilson-Barnett, J. (1979) *Stress in hospital*. Edinburgh: Churchill Livingstone.

Wolf, P. A. *et al.* (1977) Epidemiology of stroke. In: *Advances in neurology*, vol. 16. ed. R. A. Thompson and J. R. Green, pp. 5–19. New York: Raven Press.

Wood, P. H. N. (1980) *International classification of impairments, disabilities and handicaps*. Geneva, World Health Organization.

Wright, W. B. and Robson, P. (1980) Crisis procedure for stroke at home. *Lancet* **ii**, 249–50.

Zarit, S. H., Reever, K. E. and Peterson, J. (1980) Relatives of the impaired elderly: correlates of feelings of burden. *Gerontologist* **20**, 649–55.

Zola, I. K. (1973) Pathways to the doctor: from person to patient. *Soc. Sci. Med.* **7**, 677–89.

Index

Printed in the United States
77779LV00005B/98